Heart Healthy Diet After 50

Discover Culinary Delights and Strategies for a Healthy Heart and Vibrant Lifestyle

Your Complete Guide with Special Bonuses

Paul Hartman - Rose Dalia

Table of Contents

Chapter 5   **105**
A 28-Day Heart-Healthy Meal Plan

Week 1: Initiating a Heart-Healthy Regimen

Week 2: Delving Deeper into Nutritional Wellness

Week 3: Celebrating Dietary Diversity

Week 4: Reinforcing Heart-Healthy Habits

Chapter 6   **107**
The Heart-Healthy Shopping Guide

Chapter 7   **111**
Measurement Conversion Table
BONUS

1. Cardiovascular Prevention Guide

2. Trackers, Logs, Planners

Conclusion   **114**

✿ HERE IS YOU FREE GIFT!

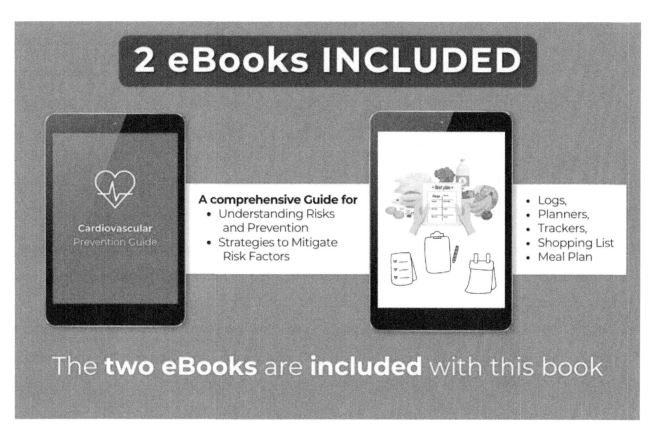

2 eBooks INCLUDED

Cardiovascular Prevention Guide

A comprehensive Guide for
- Understanding Risks and Prevention
- Strategies to Mitigate Risk Factors

- Logs,
- Planners,
- Trackers,
- Shopping List
- Meal Plan

The **two eBooks** are **included** with this book

☞ SCAN HERE TO DOWNLOAD IT

SCAN ME

Introduction

The heart, a vital organ in the human body, necessitates meticulous care and attention, particularly regarding dietary choices. In an era where heart disease is alarmingly prevalent, largely due to modern lifestyles and dietary habits, understanding the impact of what we consume is more crucial than ever. This guide is designed to be your companion in making heart-conscious culinary choices, offering a plethora of recipes that are not only delectable but also conducive to maintaining a robust heart.

Embarking on a journey towards heart-healthy eating can be a transformative experience. This cookbook is an excellent starting point for enhancing heart health through informed dietary choices. It's important to remember that change doesn't happen overnight. By making incremental, heart-healthy choices in your diet, you'll gradually notice significant improvements in your overall health. Adhering to a new eating regimen can be challenging, but the guidance provided in this book aims to ease that transition.

A heart-healthy diet is diverse and balanced, encompassing a variety of nourishing foods. It should include abundant fresh and starchy vegetables, fresh fruits, low-fat and non-fat dairy products, whole grains, lean meats, healthy fats and oils, skinless poultry, and various legumes, nuts, and seeds. These ingredients are nutritious and offer a range of flavors and textures to keep your meals interesting and enjoyable.

Coronary heart disease, the most common type of heart ailment, is a leading cause of death in the United States, often leading to strokes or heart attacks. The good news is that the power to improve your heart health lies in your hands. By making conscious choices to protect your heart, you can significantly reduce the risk of heart-related complications and ensure a longer, healthier life.

This cookbook emphasizes three major healthy eating patterns: the DASH diet, vegetarian/vegan diets, and the Mediterranean diet. Each of these diets has been shown to have significant benefits for heart health. By following the recipes and guidelines in this book, you'll enjoy delicious meals and embrace a diet that's a powerful tool against heart disease.

In addition to recipes, this guide offers insights into various nutritional aspects and lifestyle choices contributing to heart health. By understanding these elements, you can avoid the pitfalls of an unhealthy lifestyle and eating habits. With each recipe and piece of advice, you're taking a step towards a healthier heart and a better quality of life.

Let's embark on this journey together, embracing the art of heart-healthy cooking and the joy of eating well for the sake of our hearts. It's time to start making those small changes that lead to big improvements in heart health. Let's get started.

The Importance of Heart Health After 50

In today's rapidly advancing world, 50 is often heralded as the new 40. With improved healthcare, better living conditions, and an increased emphasis on wellness, people live longer and more fulfilling lives. However, as we celebrate these milestones, it's crucial to address the silent epidemic that looms large for this age group: cardiovascular diseases (CVDs).

The age of 50 is not just a numerical milestone but a significant juncture in one's physiological journey. As the body matures, it undergoes various changes, and the heart, a pivotal organ, is no exception. The heart's ability to pump blood efficiently, its rhythm, and even the health of the blood vessels can transform. These changes, while natural, can predispose an individual to a range of heart-related ailments.

Recent epidemiological data paints a concerning picture. The World Health Organization (WHO) reports that CVDs are the number one cause of death globally. More alarmingly, a significant proportion of these deaths occur in individuals aged above 50. This age group, which often stands at the cusp of retirement and looks forward to golden years filled with travel, family time, and leisure, grapples with heart health challenges.

But why is the heart particularly vulnerable after 50? The reasons are manifold. For starters, the heart muscles tend to become less elastic with age. This reduced elasticity can impair the heart's ability to pump blood, leading to conditions like heart failure. The arteries, responsible for carrying oxygen-rich blood from the heart to various parts of the body, can become stiffer and narrower due to the buildup of fatty deposits. This condition, known as atherosclerosis, can significantly increase the risk of heart attacks.

Furthermore, the factors of risk for heart diseases, such as high blood pressure, diabetes, and high cholesterol, become more prevalent as one age. Lifestyle factors, accumulated over decades, play a significant role here. A diet rich in saturated fats, sedentary habits, excessive smoking, and alcohol consumption can all take their toll on heart health.

However, it's not all gloom and doom. The silver lining in this scenario is the power of awareness and proactive intervention. Recognizing the importance of heart health after 50 is the first step towards prevention. Regular health check-ups, blood pressure and cholesterol levels monitoring, and an emphasis on a balanced diet and physical activity can go a long way in ensuring heart wellness.

Moreover, the medical community's advancements have equipped us with many tools to combat heart ailments. From state-of-the-art diagnostic tools to groundbreaking treatments, the arsenal against CVDs is robust and ever-evolving.

In conclusion, while age 50 brings certain vulnerabilities related to heart health, it also offers an opportunity. An opportunity to recalibrate, reassess, and realign one's lifestyle choices. With the right knowledge, proactive measures, and a heart-centric approach to wellness, the years post-50 can be golden, both in spirit and health.

Understanding the Aging Heart

The heart, a marvel of biological engineering, beats approximately 100,000 times daily, pumping blood throughout our body. But like all machinery, tear, and wear are inevitable. As we cross the threshold of 50, our heart undergoes a series of transformations. Understanding these changes is not just a matter of scientific curiosity; it's a call to action, a beckoning to adapt and evolve with our aging hearts.

The aging process brings many physiological changes, and the cardiovascular system is no exception. As decades pass, the very fabric of our heart, the myocardium, undergoes subtle shifts. The heart walls, especially the left ventricle, may thicken, reducing the chamber's size and blood-holding capacity. This hypertrophy, while a natural response to the increased workload and arterial stiffness, can compromise the heart's efficiency.

Arterial health is another area of concern. With age, our arteries, the highways of our circulatory system, can lose their elasticity. This arterial stiffening, often exacerbated by atherosclerotic changes, can increase blood pressure, a formidable risk factor for cardiovascular diseases. The valves within the heart, responsible for directing blood flow, may also become thicker and stiffer, leading to conditions like valvular heart disease.

Moreover, the heart's electrical system, the intricate network that ensures each heartbeat is timely and coordinated, can also show signs of aging. This can manifest as arrhythmias or irregular heart rhythms, which, while often benign, can sometimes lead to more severe complications.

However, the narrative of the aging heart is not just a tale of structural changes. It's a chronicle of resilience and adaptability. The heart's ability to increase its output during periods of stress or exercise, termed cardiac reserve, might diminish with age. Yet, the heart compensates through various mechanisms, ensuring our tissues receive oxygen and nutrients.

While these changes paint a picture of inevitable decline, it's crucial to note that not all aging hearts walk the same path. Genetics, environmental factors, and lifestyle choices play a significant role in determining how our heart ages. A sedentary lifestyle, diets rich in processed foods, smoking, and uncontrolled hypertension can accelerate the aging process. Conversely, regular exercise, a balanced diet, and timely medical interventions can act as the elixir of youth for the heart.

In the age of information, understanding the aging heart is not just the prerogative of the medical community. It's a shared responsibility. Each heartbeat and pulsation is a testament to our heart's unwavering commitment to sustaining life. As we stand at the crossroads of middle age, armed with knowledge and insights, we can shape the narrative of our aging hearts.

In essence, understanding the aging heart is akin to reading a biography filled with tales of challenges and triumphs. It's a journey that beckons us to delve deeper, appreciate the intricacies, and adapt with grace and determination. For in the heart's rhythmic beats lies the timeless saga of life itself.

Chapter #1: The Aging Heart: Insights and Implications

The heart, often symbolized as the essence of human emotion and life, undergoes a profound journey as we age. This chapter delves deep into the intricacies of the aging heart, unraveling its mysteries and highlighting the imperative of understanding its evolution.

1.1. Age-Related Changes in the Heart

Age-Related Changes in the Heart: A Deep Dive into the Heart's Evolution

As the adage goes, with age comes wisdom. But age also brings about inevitable changes in our bodies, and the heart, as our vital life pump, is no exception. Understanding the age-related transformations in the heart is crucial, not just for medical professionals but for anyone past the age of 50. This knowledge empowers individuals to make informed decisions about their health, leading to a better quality of life.

Structural Transformations

One of the most pronounced changes the heart undergoes with age is its structure. Over time, the heart walls, especially the left ventricle, tend to thicken. This thickening, known as hypertrophy, can compensate for the increased workload or high blood pressure. While it might sound beneficial, this adaptation can reduce the heart's efficiency, making it harder to fill with blood and pump it out.

Moreover, the chambers of the heart, which hold and pump blood, may reduce in size. This reduction can decrease cardiac output, meaning the heart pumps less blood each beat. Over time, this can lead to fatigue and shortness of breath, particularly during physical activities.

Arterial and Valvular Health

The heart is intricately connected to a network of veins and arteries. With age, these arteries lose some of their elasticity, becoming stiffer. This loss of flexibility can increase the risk of high blood pressure, as the arteries resist the blood flow. Furthermore, atherosclerotic changes, characterized by the buildup of fatty plaques in the arteries, can begin to manifest. These plaques can constrict the arteries, reducing blood flow and potentially leading to heart attacks.

The heart valves, which ensure the unidirectional blood flow, also change. They can become thicker and stiffer, leading to conditions like valvular stenosis or regurgitation. In simple terms, the valves don't open or close as they should, which can disrupt the normal flow of blood.

The Heart's Electrical System

A complex electrical system orchestrates the heart's rhythm. As we age, changes in this system can lead to irregular heart rhythms or arrhythmias. Some of these irregularities are benign, but others can be life-threatening. For instance, atrial fibrillation, a common arrhythmia in older people, can increase the risk of stroke.

Age-induced alterations in the heart's electrical network can manifest as slower heart rates or blocked electrical pathways. These changes can sometimes necessitate interventions like pacemaker implantations to maintain a regular heart rhythm.

In conclusion, the heart's evolution with age is a testament to the body's adaptability. However, these changes also highlight the importance of a proactive approach to heart health and regular medical check-ups. By understanding the transformations our hearts undergo, we can better appreciate the need for a heart-healthy lifestyle, timely medical interventions, and the importance of staying informed. After all, knowledge, when applied, is the first line of defense against the challenges that age presents to our cardiac well-being.

1.2. Prevalent Heart Conditions After 50

The golden years post-50 bring many experiences, memories, and wisdom. However, they also usher in an increased susceptibility to certain health conditions, especially heart-related ones. As we age, our cardiovascular system faces challenges that can lead to various heart conditions. Recognizing and understanding these conditions is the first step towards proactive management and ensuring a heart-healthy life.

Coronary Artery Disease (CAD)

Arguably the most common heart-related ailment in those over 50, CAD, happens when the coronary arteries, responsible for supplying blood to the heart muscle, become narrowed or blocked due to a buildup of cholesterol-laden plaques. This can lead to a heart attack or chest pain (angina). Lifestyle factors such as diet, exercise, smoking, and stress play a significant role in the development and progression of CAD.

Heart Failure

Often misunderstood as a condition where the heart stops working entirely, heart failure refers to the heart's inability to pump blood efficiently to meet the body's needs. This can result from conditions that have weakened the heart or made it stiff. Symptoms include fatigue, shortness of breath, and swelling in the legs and abdomen.

Atrial Fibrillation (AFib)

AFib is an irregular, often rapid heart rate that can lead to stroke and other heart-related complications. It's characterized by the two upper chambers of the heart (the atria) beating chaotically and out of sync with the two lower chambers (the ventricles). This arrhythmia becomes more common with age and can result from high blood pressure, CAD, or valve disorders.

Valvular Heart Diseases

Age can take a toll on the heart valves, leading to conditions like aortic stenosis (narrowing of the aortic valve), mitral regurgitation (backward flow of blood due to a leaky mitral valve), or aortic regurgitation (leakage of the aortic valve). These conditions can cause symptoms ranging from shortness of breath to fainting spells.

Peripheral Artery Disease (PAD)

While not a condition of the heart per se, PAD is closely related to heart health. It occurs when the peripheral arteries, mainly those supplying blood to the legs, narrow. It's often a sign of widespread accumulation of fatty deposits in the arteries, which may reduce blood flow to the heart and brain.

Cardiomyopathy

Cardiomyopathy refers to diseases of the heart muscle. In cardiomyopathy, the heart muscle becomes thick, enlarged, or rigid; in rare cases, muscle tissue is replaced with scar tissue. As the condition worsens, the heart becomes weaker and less able to pump blood effectively.

High Blood Pressure (Hypertension)

Often dubbed the "silent killer" because it can exist without any clear symptoms, hypertension can lead to both heart and kidney diseases. Especially after 50, regular monitoring is crucial to ensure that blood pressure remains within a healthy range.

In conclusion, the post-50 phase of life requires a heightened awareness of heart health. While age-related changes in the heart are natural, the onset of heart conditions can often be managed or even prevented with timely interventions, regular check-ups, and lifestyle modifications. Knowledge of these prevalent conditions is not just power; it's a roadmap to a healthier heart and a longer, more fulfilling life.

1.3. The Genetic Landscape and Familial Predispositions

The intricate tapestry of our genetic makeup holds clues to our past, present, and future health. When it comes to heart health, understanding the genetic landscape and familial predispositions becomes paramount, especially as we navigate the years beyond 50. Delving into the genetic underpinnings of heart health can offer insights into risks, prevention, and tailored interventions.

The Role of Genetics in Heart Health

Every individual inherits genes from their parents, which determine various characteristics, from eye color to certain health risks. Some genes, or combinations, can increase the likelihood of developing specific heart conditions. For instance, certain genetic mutations can lead to cardiomyopathies, conditions where the heart muscle becomes enlarged or thickened.

Familial Hypercholesterolemia (FH)

FH is a prime example of a genetic condition that affects heart health. It's an inherited disorder characterized by higher cholesterol levels in the blood, specifically low-density lipoprotein (LDL) cholesterol. Individuals with FH have a higher risk of developing coronary artery disease at a younger age because of prolonged exposure to high cholesterol levels.

Familial Predispositions and Shared Environment

While genetics play a crucial role, it's essential to differentiate between purely genetic predispositions and shared familial environmental factors. Families often share diets, lifestyles, and habits, which can influence heart health. For instance, a family with a history of heart disease might also have a tradition of high-fat diets or sedentary lifestyles, both of which contribute to heart risks.

Genetic Testing and Heart Health

With advancements in medical technology, genetic testing has become more accessible. Such tests can identify mutations joined to certain heart conditions. For example, individuals with a family history of sudden cardiac deaths might undergo genetic testing to determine if they carry mutations associated with arrhythmogenic disorders.

The Power of Foreknowledge

Understanding one's genetic predisposition to heart conditions can be empowering. It allows individuals to take proactive measures, from lifestyle changes to medical interventions, to mitigate risks. Regular screenings, tailored dietary plans, and specific medications can be more effectively administered when one is aware of their genetic landscape.

The Ethical Dimension

While genetic insights offer a wealth of information, they also bring ethical considerations. Knowing a genetic predisposition can lead to anxiety or affect life choices. Moreover, there's the question of privacy and the potential misuse of genetic data. Individuals must be counseled appropriately before and after undergoing genetic testing.

A Holistic Approach to Heart Health

While genetics provide a piece of the puzzle, heart health is multifaceted. Environmental factors, lifestyle choices, and random events determine heart health outcomes. A balanced diet, regular exercise, stress management, and regular medical check-ups remain the pillars of heart health, regardless of one's genetic makeup.

In conclusion, exploring the genetic landscape and familial predispositions offers a deeper understanding of heart health, especially as we age. It underscores the interconnectedness of genes, environment, and choices. By embracing the knowledge genetics offers and combining it with proactive health measures, individuals can chart a course towards optimal heart health, armed with the insights of both their inherited blueprint and the choices they make in life.

Chapter #2: Fundamentals of a Heart-Healthy Diet

As we age, our bodies undergo many changes, directly impacting our nutritional needs and how our bodies process food. Understanding these shifts is crucial for maintaining optimal health and preventing age-related diseases, especially those concerning the heart.

2.1. Nutritional Considerations for the Aging Population

Changing Metabolic Rates

One of the most significant changes that occur with age is the slowing down our metabolism. This natural decline means that our bodies require fewer calories as we age. However, this doesn't mean that our need for essential nutrients decreases. The demand for certain nutrients, such as calcium and vitamin D, may increase. This poses a challenge: how does one meet their nutritional needs without excess calories? The answer lies in opting for nutrient-dense foods that provide a high level of vitamins and minerals relative to their caloric content. Examples include leafy greens, berries, and lean proteins.

Nutrient Absorption and Digestion

Age can also impact the efficiency of our digestive system. The body's ability to absorb certain nutrients, such as vitamin B12, can diminish. This is due to decreased stomach acid production, essential for B12 absorption. Moreover, atrophic gastritis, common in older adults, can further reduce stomach acid production. Older adults might benefit from consuming fortified foods or supplements to combat this.

Bone Health and Calcium Needs

Bone density naturally decreases as we age, leading to conditions like osteoporosis, which can increase the risk of fractures. While this might not seem directly related to heart health, there's a connection. Some studies suggest that bone and heart health are intertwined, possibly due to shared regulatory mechanisms involving calcium and vitamin D. Ensuring an adequate intake of these nutrients is crucial. While dairy is a well-known source of calcium, other foods like fortified plant-based milk, green leafy vegetables, and fish-like sardines are excellent sources.

Hydration and Electrolyte Balance

Hydration is a key component of overall health, but its importance is often overlooked in older adults. With age, the sensation of thirst may diminish, leading to reduced fluid intake. Dehydration can have severe consequences, including a rising risk of urinary tract infections, kidney stones, and chronic kidney disease. Besides, also, as well, dehydration can lead to an imbalance in electrolytes, which play a crucial role in heart function. Maintaining hydration is not just about drinking water; it's also about consuming foods with high water content, such as vegetables and fruits.

In conclusion, understanding the unique nutritional needs and challenges the aging population faces is essential for promoting heart health and overall well-being. While age might bring about certain limitations, it also offers the wisdom to make informed and health-conscious decisions. By focusing on nutrient-dense foods, staying hydrated, and being aware of the body's changing needs, older adults can pave the way for a heart-healthy future.

2.2. Dietary Components to Prioritise

The foods we consume are pivotal in achieving and maintaining heart health, especially as we age. While it's essential to be aware of what to avoid, knowing which dietary components should take precedence in our meals is equally crucial. Prioritizing these elements can significantly reduce the risk of heart disease and promote overall well-being.

Omega-3 Fatty Acids

Omega-3 fatty acids, particularly those in fatty fish like sardines, mackerel, and salmon, have been lauded for their heart-protective properties. These fats help reduce inflammation, lower the risk of arrhythmias (abnormal heartbeats), and decrease triglyceride levels. Walnuts, flaxseeds, and chia seeds are excellent plant-based sources for those who don't consume fish.

Dietary Fiber

Fiber is a heart's best friend. It is found abundantly in whole grains, fruits, vegetables, and legumes; dietary fiber can help lower bad cholesterol levels, thus reducing the risk of heart disease. Additionally, fiber aids in achieving a feeling of fullness, which can avoid overeating and assist in weight management, a crucial aspect of heart health.

Antioxidants and Phytonutrients

Brightly colored fruits and vegetables are packed with antioxidants and phytonutrients. These compounds help combat oxidative stress in the body, which can damage cells and increase the risk of heart disease. Berries, tomatoes, broccoli, nuts, and seeds are just a few foods rich in these protective compounds.

Potassium

Potassium is an essential mineral that is vigorous in maintaining proper heart function. It helps regulate blood pressure by neutralizing the effects of sodium and reducing tension in the blood vessel walls. Potassium-rich foods include bananas, oranges, cantaloupes, spinach, beans, and potatoes.

Magnesium

Magnesium is another mineral that deserves attention when prioritizing heart health. It's involved in over 300 enzymatic reactions in the body, including those that regulate heart rhythm. Magnesium can be found in almonds, cashews, black beans, and whole grains.

Plant Sterols and Stanols

Plant sterols and stanols are naturally occurring substances found in plants that help lower cholesterol levels. They work by blocking the absorption of cholesterol in the intestines. While they are found in small amounts in fruits, vegetables, and grains, many products are now fortified for added heart health benefits.

Lean Proteins

Prioritizing lean proteins over fatty cuts of meat can significantly benefit the heart. Poultry, lean beef, tofu, and legumes are excellent protein sources without the added saturated fats that can elevate cholesterol levels.

Healthy Fats

While it's essential to reduce the intake of saturated and trans fats, it's equally important to ensure an adequate intake of healthy fats. Avocados, olive oil, nuts, and seeds provide monounsaturated and polyunsaturated fats that can improve heart health by reducing bad cholesterol levels and providing essential nutrients.

In conclusion, prioritizing these dietary components can pave the way for a heart-healthy lifestyle. It's about restriction and making informed choices that nourish the body and support cardiovascular function. Individuals can take proactive steps towards a healthier heart and a longer, more vibrant life by focusing on these essential nutrients and foods.

2.3. Foods with Potential Cardiac Risks

In the journey towards achieving optimal heart health, it's not just about knowing what to eat but also what to limit or avoid. While food with potential cardiac risks might be tantalizing to the taste buds, certain foods can pose significant risks to the heart, especially when consumed in excess. Recognizing these potential threats is crucial for anyone aiming to maintain a heart-healthy lifestyle, particularly as they age.

Processed Meat

Deli meats, bacon, sausages, and hot dogs might be convenient and delicious, but they come with a hefty dose of sodium, preservatives, and unhealthy fats. Regular consumption of these processed meats has been linked to an increased risk of heart disease, high blood pressure, and certain types of cancer.

Sugary Beverages

Sodas, sweetened teas, and other sugary drinks might quench your thirst, but they can wreak havoc on heart health. High sugar intake can lead to weight gain, increased risk of type 2 diabetes, and elevated triglyceride levels, all of which are risk factors for heart disease.

Trans Fats

Often found in margarine, snack foods, baked goods, and fried foods, trans fats are a major culprit in raising LDL (bad) cholesterol levels while lowering HDL (good) cholesterol. This double setback can significantly increase the risk of heart disease.

Excessive Salt

While sodium is essential for bodily functions, excessive salt intake is a leading cause of high blood pressure, a major risk factor for heart disease and stroke. Processed foods, canned soups, and certain restaurant dishes can be surprisingly high in sodium.

Refined Carbohydrates and Sugars: White bread, pastries, and other foods made with refined carbohydrates can cause rapid spikes in blood sugar, leading to insulin resistance over time. This can pave the way for type 2 diabetes, a known risk factor for heart disease.

Alcohol

While moderate alcohol consumption might offer some heart benefits, excessive drinking can lead to high blood pressure, heart failure, and stroke. Moreover, alcohol is calorie-dense, contributing to weight gain, a risk factor for heart disease.

Deep-Fried Food

Deep-fried foods, especially in unhealthy oils, contain calories and trans fats. Regular consumption can lead to weight gain, increased cholesterol levels, and high blood pressure, all of which strain the heart.

Commercially Baked Goods

Muffins, donuts, and cookies from commercial sources often contain trans fats, refined sugar, and other unhealthy ingredients. These can elevate cholesterol, promote inflammation, and increase the risk of heart disease.

Certain Dairy Products

While dairy can be part of a balanced diet, full-fat versions like whole milk, butter, and cheese are high in saturated fats. These can raise LDL cholesterol levels, increasing the risk of heart disease.

Caffeine Overload

While a cup of coffee can offer antioxidants, excessive caffeine can lead to irregular heart rhythms and high blood pressure. It's essential to consume it in moderation.

In conclusion, while occasionally indulging in foods with potential cardiac risks is part of life, it's vital to be aware of the potential cardiac risks associated with certain foods. Individuals can significantly reduce their risk of heart-related ailments by making informed dietary choices and prioritizing heart-healthy alternatives. It's not about deprivation but about understanding the implications of our choices and striving for a balanced, heart-conscious diet.

Chapter #3: Diet and Cardiovascular Health: The Underlying Connections

Understanding the intricate relationship between diet and heart health is pivotal. The foods we consume directly impact various cardiovascular parameters, influencing our overall heart health. This chapter delves deep into the connections, shedding light on the implications of cholesterol, the challenges posed by hypertension, and the effects of processed foods and sugars on the cardiovascular system.

3.1. Cholesterol: Implications for Cardiac Health

Cholesterol, a waxy, fat-like substance, is a crucial component of every cell in our body. It aids in producing essential hormones, vitamin D, and substances that help digest food. However, when present in excessive amounts in the bloodstream, cholesterol can harm cardiac health.

The Basics of Cholesterol

Cholesterol doesn't travel alone in the bloodstream. It pairs with proteins, forming lipoproteins. The density of these lipoproteins determines their classification:

1) High-Density Lipoprotein (HDL): Often termed the 'good' cholesterol, HDL carries cholesterol away from the arteries to the liver, where it's processed and expelled from the body. High levels of HDL are associated with a reduced risk of heart disease

2) Low-Density Lipoprotein (LDL): The 'bad' cholesterol transports cholesterol particles throughout the body. High levels of LDL can lead to the build-up of cholesterol in the arteries, initiating atherosclerosis, a precursor to heart disease.

3) Triglycerides are another type of fat in the blood that can increase the risk of heart disease when elevated.

Dietary Sources of Cholesterol

Historically, dietary cholesterol, found in animal products like meat, dairy, and eggs, was believed to be a primary culprit in raising blood cholesterol. However, recent research suggests that the cholesterol ingested from food minimizes blood cholesterol for most people.

Instead, saturated and trans fats have a more significant impact on blood cholesterol levels.

The Cholesterol-Heart Disease Link

Too much LDL cholesterol in the blood can get deposited on the walls of the arteries, leading to the formation of plaques. These plaques narrow the arteries, reducing blood flow to the heart muscle. Over time, blockages can form, increasing the risk of heart attack or stroke.

Furthermore, when these plaques rupture, they can trigger a blood clot, blocking the flow of blood and leading to acute cardiac events. Elevated cholesterol, especially LDL, is a significant risk factor for coronary heart disease, heart attack, and stroke.

Foods that Help Regulate Cholesterol

Certain foods can actively help in reducing cholesterol levels:

- Oats and Whole Grains: Rich in soluble fiber, they can lower LDL cholesterol.
- Fatty Fish: Sardines, mackerel, and salmon are high in omega-3 fatty acids, which can reduce overall cholesterol.
- Nuts: Almonds and walnuts can reduce blood cholesterol. They contain high amounts of unsaturated fats, which benefit the heart.
- Olive Oil: Contains antioxidants that can lower LDL while leaving HDL untouched.

The Role of Medication and Lifestyle

For individuals who can't manage their cholesterol through diet and exercise alone, medications might be necessary. Statins are the most common cholesterol-lowering drugs. However, pairing medication with lifestyle changes is crucial for optimal heart health.

In conclusion, while cholesterol is essential for various bodily functions, its excessive presence in the bloodstream can harm heart health. Understanding cholesterol and its implications is the first step in managing and optimizing cardiac health.

3.2. Hypertension: The Unspoken Cardiovascular Challenge

Hypertension, commonly known as high blood pressure, is a silent yet potent threat to cardiovascular health. Often going unnoticed due to its asymptomatic nature, it's a primary or contributing cause of nearly half a million deaths annually. Understanding hypertension, its implications, and management is crucial in the fight against cardiovascular diseases.

Understanding Blood Pressure Metrics

Blood pressure is the force exerted by circulating blood against the walls of the body's arteries. Two measurements denote it:

- Systolic Pressure: The higher number representing the force exerted when the heart contracts and pumps blood into the arteries.
- Diastolic Pressure: The lower number indicates the pressure when the heart rests between beats.

A normal reading is characteristic of around 120/80 mm Hg. Hypertension is diagnosed when blood pressure readings exceed 140/90 mm Hg.

Causes and Risk Factors

While the exact causes of hypertension aren't always clear, several factors and conditions may increase the risk:

- Age: The risk of hypertension increases as you age.
- Family History: It often runs in families.
- Tobacco Use: Smoking or chewing tobacco increases blood pressure.
- Dietary Choices: High salt intake, low potassium diet, and excessive alcohol can elevate blood pressure levels.
- Physical Inactivity: A sedentary lifestyle increases heart rate, leading to higher pressure on arteries.
- Obesity: More blood is needed to supply oxygen and nutrients to tissues in excess-weight individuals, increasing the pressure on artery walls.

Hypertension's Impact on Cardiovascular Health

Unchecked hypertension can lead to severe health complications:

- Atherosclerosis: High pressure can cause arteries to narrow and harden, leading to this condition, resulting in heart disease or stroke.
- Heart Enlargement or Failure to pump blood against the higher pressure in the vessels, the heart must work harder, which can cause it to enlarge and fail to supply blood to the body adequately.
- Kidney Damage: The kidneys' filtering system relies on a dense network of blood vessels. Expected time, high blood pressure can narrow and thicken these vessels.

Managing Hypertension

While hypertension poses significant risks, it's manageable with the right approach:

- Dietary Changes: A diet rich in whole grains, fruits, vegetables, and low-fat dairy products can significantly lower blood pressure. Reducing sodium intake is also crucial.
- Physical Activity: Regular exercise strengthens the heart, allowing it to pump more blood with less effort, reducing the force on arteries.

- Medication: For many, lifestyle changes aren't enough. Blood pressure medications come in various classes, each with its mechanism of action.
- Limiting Alcohol and Caffeine: Both can raise blood pressure. It's essential to consume them in moderation.
- Stress Management: Chronic stress can contribute to hypertension. Finding healthy ways to manage stress, such as meditation, deep breathing exercises, and physical activity, can be beneficial.

In conclusion, hypertension, often dubbed the "silent killer," is a significant cardiovascular challenge due to its stealthy nature. Regular monitoring, understanding the risks, and proactive management can mitigate its adverse effects, ensuring a healthier heart and longer life.

3.3. Processed Foods and Sugars: A Closer Examination

In today's fast-paced world, the convenience of processed foods is undeniable. These products dominate supermarket shelves and our diets, from ready-to-eat meals to sugary beverages. However, the implications of their consumption, especially concerning cardiovascular health, warrant a closer look.

What Are Processed Foods?

Processed foods have undergone changes from their natural state for convenience, longevity, or taste purposes. These changes can involve smoking, salting, fermenting, canning, or adding preservatives. While not all processed foods are harmful, many contain unhealthy fats, salt, and sugar.

The Sugar Surge

Sugar, particularly added sugars, is a primary concern in processed foods. These aren't the sugars naturally found in fruits or milk but those added during processing or preparation. Common culprits include sodas, candies, baked goods, and many so-called "low-fat" foods.

Implications for Cardiovascular Health

- Inflammation: High sugar intake can lead to inflammation, a root cause of various chronic diseases, including heart diseases. Inflammation can damage arteries, leading to chronic conditions like atherosclerosis.
- Weight Gain: Processed foods, especially those high in sugars and unhealthy fats, are calorie-dense. Regular consumption can lead to weight gain, a significant risk factor for heart disease
- High Blood Pressure: Many processed foods contain excessive salt, contributing to hypertension, a leading cause of cardiovascular diseases.
- Disruption in Blood Lipids: High intake of processed foods can increase LDL (bad cholesterol) and decrease HDL (good cholesterol), leading to plaque buildup in arteries.
- Insulin Resistance: Excessive sugar consumption can lead to insulin resistance, a precursor to type 2 diabetes, which is closely linked to heart disease.

The Hidden Dangers of Sugary Beverages

Sugary drinks, including sodas, sweet teas, and even fruit drinks, are among the diet's most significant sources of added sugars. Regular consumption is linked to obesity, type 2 diabetes, and, consequently, increased heart disease risk.

Decoding Labels: The Challenge of Hidden Sugars

One of the challenges consumers face is the myriad of names sugar hides under in ingredient lists. Fructose, high fructose corn syrup, cane sugar, maltose, dextrose, and beet sugar are just a few. Being aware of these names can help in making informed choices.

Making Healthier Choices

- Read Labels: Always check the nutrition label. Look for foods with fewer ingredients, low added sugars, and minimal saturated fats.
- Opt for Natural: Choose whole foods like fresh fruits, vegetables, lean meats, and whole grains over processed alternatives.
- Limit Sugary Beverages: Opt for water, unsweetened teas, or beverages without added sugars.
- Cook at Home: Preparing meals at home allows control over ingredients, ensuring a heart-healthy diet.
- Educate and Advocate: The first step is to be informed about the risks of processed foods and sugars. Sharing this knowledge with loved ones can create a ripple effect, promoting community health.

In conclusion, while processed foods offer convenience, their potential impact on heart health is concerning. By understanding the risks, reading labels, and making informed dietary choices, enjoying a diet that supports cardiovascular health without sacrificing taste or convenience is possible.

Chapter #4: Culinary Delights for a Healthy Heart

The heart is not just an organ; it's the very essence of life. And what better way to care for it than through the foods we consume? This chapter delves deep into the culinary world, offering many heart-healthy recipes that don't compromise on taste.

4.1. Breakfast Selections for a Heart-Healthy Start

1. Zucchini Stuffed Breakfast

Preparation time: 10 minutes

Cooking time: 15 minutes

Serving: 2

Difficulty level: Easy

Ingredients

- 6 zucchinis (approximately 1.2 kg or 2.65 lbs)
- 3/4 cup shredded mozzarella cheese (approx. 86 g or 3 oz)
- 3/4 cup cooked turkey breast, diced (approx. 113 g or 4 oz)
- 1/4 tsp black pepper (approx. 0.5 g)
- 2 medium tomatoes, diced (approx. 180 g or 6.3 oz)
- 2 tbsp fresh basil, chopped (approx. 5.3 g or 0.19 oz)
- 1/2 cup panko breadcrumbs (approx. 60 g or 2.1 oz)
- 2 tbsp fresh oregano, chopped (approx. 5.3 g or 0.19 oz)
- 1/3 cup grated parmesan cheese (approx. 30 g or 1 oz)
- 1/3 cup fresh parsley, chopped (approx. 15 g or 0.5 oz)
- Oil for brushing (quantity as needed)

Directions:

1. Preheat the oven to 350°F (175°C). Lightly oil a baking sheet. Halve the zucchinis lengthwise, scoop out the pulp to create a hollow, and chop the pulp finely. Place the zucchini halves on the prepared baking sheet.
2. Over medium heat, cook the diced turkey breast in a skillet until browned, about 4 minutes.
3. Remove the skillet from heat. Add the chopped zucchini pulp, diced tomatoes, shredded mozzarella, grated parmesan, panko breadcrumbs, chopped basil, oregano, parsley, and black pepper to the turkey. Mix well to combine.
4. Spoon the mixture into the hollowed zucchini halves. Bake in the oven until the zucchini is tender, and the topping is golden brown, about 15 minutes.

Nutritional information

- *Calories: 180 kcal*
- *Total Fat: 5.2 g / 0,17 oz*
- *Protein: 23.5 g / 0,84*
- *Carbohydrates: 10 g / 0,35*
- *Sodium: 35 mg / 0,001 oz*

---

2. Green Scrambled Eggs

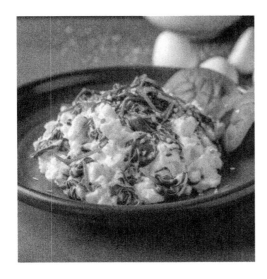

Preparation time: 10 minutes

Cooking time: 30 minutes

Serving: 2

Difficulty level: Medium

Ingredients

- 4 large eggs
- 1/4 tsp salt (1.5 g / 0.053 oz)
- 1/4 tsp black pepper (0.5 g / 0.018 oz)
- 2 tsp unsalted butter (9.4 g / 0.33 oz)
- A handful of arugula leaves, chopped (about 1 cup or 20 g / 0.7 oz)

- 8 cherry tomatoes, halved (about 150 g / 5.3 oz)
- 1/4 cup chopped roasted red peppers, no added salt (about 54 g / 1.9 oz)
- 1 avocado, peeled, pitted, and diced (about 150 g / 5.3 oz)

Directions:

1. In a bowl, crack the eggs. Season with black pepper and salt, then whisk thoroughly.
2. In a nonstick skillet, melt the butter over medium-low heat.
3. Once the butter begins to froth, introduce the arugula/spinach and sauté for about a minute.
4. Transfer the sautéed arugula/spinach onto a plate.
5. Pour the whisked eggs into the skillet, stirring occasionally to scramble.
6. As the eggs near completion, sprinkle in the tomatoes, previously sautéed arugula/spinach, and red pepper. Refrain from stirring.
7. Place the lid on the skillet and allow it to cook for an additional minute.
8. Garnish with the diced avocado.

Nutritional information

- *Calories: 538 kcal*
- *Total Fat: 33.6 g / 1,13 oz*
- *Sodium: 842 mg / 0,02 oz*
- *Carbohydrates: 38.8 g / 1,40 oz*
- *Protein: 21 g / 0,74*

3. Roasted Pepper Frittata

Preparation time: 15 minutes

Cooking time: 24 minutes

Serving: 2

Difficulty level: Easy

Ingredients

- 2 tbsp (tablespoons) olive oil
- 1/2 cup (approximately 75 g - 2,5 oz) chopped onions
- 8 large eggs, beaten
- 1/4 tsp (teaspoon) black pepper
- 3 cups (approximately 90 g - 3 oz) roughly chopped spinach
- 1/2 cup (approximately 75 g - 2,5 oz) roughly chopped simple roasted peppers
- 1/3 cup (approximately 50 g - 1,7 oz) crumbled feta cheese

Directions:

1. Preheat the oven to 350°F (approximately 175°C).
2. Heat the olive oil over medium-high heat in an 8- to 10-inch oven-safe skillet. Once hot, introduce the onions and sauté until they soften, which should take around 5 minutes.
3. In a separate bowl, whisk together the eggs and black pepper.
4. Add the chopped spinach to the skillet, allowing it to wilt slightly over 1 to 2 minutes.
5. Incorporate the red peppers, continuing to sauté for 1 to 2 minutes.
6. Reduce the heat to medium and pour the beaten eggs, stirring briefly to ensure even distribution.
7. Sprinkle the crumbled feta cheese atop the mixture.
8. Transfer the skillet to the oven and bake until the eggs have set, which should be approximately 15 minutes.

Nutritional information

- *Calories: 253 kcal*
- *Total Fat: 20.1 g / 0,70 oz*
- *Sodium: 322 mg / 0,011 oz*
- *Carbohydrates: 4 g / 0,14 oz*
- *Protein: 15.3 g / 0,50 oz*

⚠ This recipe contains feta cheese, which can be high in sodium. Those with hypertension or other heart conditions should choose a low-sodium cheese alternative. Recommendation: To reduce fat content, use fewer yolks and more egg whites.

4. Spinach Burrito

Preparation time: 5 minutes

Cooking time: 25 minutes

Serving: 2

Difficulty level: Hard

Ingredients

- 3 large eggs
- 2 whole-grain tortillas (10-inch diameter each)
- 4 thin slices of cheddar cheese
- 2 cups (approximately 60 g or 2 oz) spinach
- 1 medium tomato, finely chopped
- 2 tbsp (tablespoons) fresh tomato salsa (about 28 grams or 1 oz)
- 1 tbsp (tablespoon) olive oil

Directions:

1. In a mixing bowl, crack open the eggs and whisk them gently using a fork.
2. Lay out 2 plates and place a tortilla on each. Align 2 slices of cheddar cheese down the center of each tortilla.
3. Layer each tortilla with an equal portion of spinach, followed by the chopped tomato and salsa.
4. Heat the olive oil over medium heat in a nonstick skillet, ensuring the pan is evenly coated.
5. Pour in the beaten eggs, stirring until they achieve a scrambled consistency.
6. Once the eggs are cooked, distribute them evenly over the tomatoes and salsa on each tortilla.
7. Carefully fold in the sides of the tortillas and roll them up to form burritos.
8. Position the burritos seam-side down in the skillet (cleaned if necessary). Cover and allow them to warm gently for approximately 2-3 minutes over medium heat.
9. Serve immediately.

Nutritional information

- *Calories: 451 kcal*
- *Total Fat: 27.9 g / 1.98 oz*
- *Sodium: 1162 mg / 1.162 g*
- *Carbohydrates: 34.1 g / 1.20 oz*
- *Protein: 20.3 g / 0.72 oz*

⚠ It is recommended to use low-sodium cheese and salsa and reduce the cheese quantity or substitute with a lower-fat option.

---

5. Trail Hot Cereal

Preparation time: 10 minutes

Cooking time: 10 minutes

Serving: 2

Difficulty level: Medium

Ingredients

- 1 cup (236.6 ml / 8.45 fl oz) hot wheat cereal
- 2 tbsp (30 ml / 1 fl oz) mixed dried fruit
- 2 tbsp (30 ml / 1 fl oz) mixed nuts, unsalted
- 2 tbsp (30 ml / 1 fl oz) ground flaxseed

Directions:

1. Begin by cooking the hot wheat cereal as per package instructions. Once cooked, transfer it to serving bowls.
2. Sprinkle each bowl with an even distribution of flaxseeds, mixed nuts, and dry fruits.
3. Serve immediately while warm.

Nutritional information

- *Calories: 227 kcal*
- *Total Fat: 11 g / 0.39 oz*
- *Carbohydrates: 28.5 g / 1.01 oz*
- *Protein: 6.3 g / 0.22 oz*
- *Sodium: 16.1 mg / 0.0161 g*

6. Breakfast Cereal with Apples and Raisins

Preparation time: 10 minutes

Cooking time:20minutes

 Serving: 2

Difficulty level: Easy

Ingredients

- 1/2 tsp (teaspoon) cinnamon
- 1/8 tsp (teaspoon) nutmeg
- 1 tbsp (tablespoon) flaxseed oil
- 2 1/2 cups (approximately 600 ml) fortified, unsweetened, low-fat almond or rice milk
- 1/2 cup (approximately 95 g - 3,35 oz) whole-grain buckwheat
- 1/4 cup (approximately 35 g - 1,20 oz) coarsely chopped apples
- 1 tbsp (tablespoon) golden raisins

Directions:

1. Pour the almond or rice milk into a skillet and bring it to a simmer over medium heat.
2. Add the buckwheat, reduce the heat to low, and let it simmer. Cook for about 10 minutes, keeping it partially covered and stirring occasionally. Remove the skillet from the heat.
3. Stir in the apples and raisins, allowing the mixture to rest for 5 minutes. Finally, blend in the nutmeg, flaxseed oil, and cinnamon.
4. Serve warm.

Nutritional information

- *Calories: 133 kcal*
- *Total Fat: 4.6 g / 0.16 oz*
- *Carbohydrates: 18.8 g / 0.66 oz*
- *Protein: 1.8 g / 0.06 oz*
- *Sodium: 89 mg / 0.089 g*

7. Greek Eggs with Potatoes

Preparation time: 10 minutes

Cooking time: 36 minutes

Serving: 2

Difficulty level: Easy

Ingredients

- 3 medium tomatoes, seeded and coarsely chopped (approximately 450 g - 15,90 oz)
- Sea salt and freshly ground pepper to taste
- 3 large russet potatoes (approximately 900 g - 31,80 oz)
- 3 large eggs
- 2 tbsp (30 ml) fresh chopped basil
- 1 garlic clove, minced
- 2 tbsp(tablespoon) (30 ml) plus 1/2 cup (120 ml) olive oil, divided
- 1 tsp (teaspoon) (5 ml) fresh oregano, chopped

Directions:

1. Puree the tomatoes using a food processor.
2. Combine garlic, basil, sea salt, 2 tbsp of olive oil, and freshly ground pepper in a large skillet. Cover the skillet over low heat, and cook for 20-25 minutes until the sauce thickens and bubbles.
3. Dice the russet potatoes into small cubes. Heat 1/2 cup of olive oil over medium-low heat in a nonstick skillet.
4. Fry the potato cubes for about 5 minutes until they turn crisp and brown. At that time, cover the skillet and reduce the heat to low.
5. Carefully crack the eggs into the tomato sauce mixture. Continue cooking over low heat for approximately 6 minutes, ensuring the eggs set within the sauce.
6. Remove the potatoes from the skillet and drain any excess oil using paper towels. Transfer the potatoes to a serving bowl.
7. Season the potatoes with sea salt freshly ground pepper, and sprinkle with oregano.
8. Carefully plate the eggs alongside the potatoes. Drizzle the tomato sauce over the top before serving.

Nutritional information

- *Calories: 930 kcal*
- *Total Fat: 67 g / 2.36 oz*
- *Carbohydrates: 73 g / 2.57 oz*
- *Protein: 12 g / 0.42 oz*
- *Sodium: 249 mg / 0.249 g*

⚠ Recommendations: (1) Reduce Oil: Consider reducing the amount of olive oil to lower the total fat content. (2) Portion Control: Serve smaller portions to decrease calorie and fat intake.

8. Delicious Breakfast Barley

Preparation time: 10 minutes

Cooking time: 30 minutes

Serving: 2

Difficulty level: Medium

Ingredients

- 1 cup (approximately 240 ml) pearl barley
- 1/4 tsp (teaspoon) ground cinnamon
- 2 tbsp (tablespoon) chopped hazelnuts
- 2 tbsp (tablespoon) sliced almonds
- 1/4 cup (approximately 60 ml) frozen strawberries
- 1/4 cup (approximately 60 ml) frozen blueberries
- 4 cups (approximately 960 ml) water
- A pinch of salt

Directions:

1. In a saucepan, combine barley, water, and salt. Bring the mixture to a boil.
2. Reduce the heat to low and let it simmer for 25-30 minutes or until the barley is fully cooked.
3. Remove the saucepan from the heat and allow the mixture to cool.
4. Incorporate the remaining ingredients into the cooled barley mixture, ensuring a thorough mix.
5. Serve immediately and savor the flavors.

Nutritional information

- *Calories: 237 kcal*
- *Total Fat: 4.4 g*
- *Carbohydrates: 44.9 g*
- *Protein: 6.7 g*

9. Peanut Butter Oats

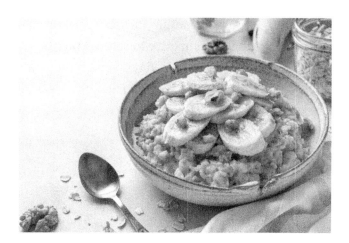

Preparation time: 5 minutes

Cooking time: 8 hours (overnight)

Serving: 2

Difficulty level: Easy

Ingredients

- 1/2 banana
- 1/2 cup (approximately 120 ml) rolled oats
- 1 tbsp (tablespoon) powdered peanut butter
- 1/2 cup (approximately 120 ml) soymilk
- 1 tbsp (tablespoon) maple syrup

- 1 tbsp (tablespoon) chia seeds
- 1/2 cup (approximately 120 ml) berries
- 1 tbsp (tablespoon) salt (adjust to taste)

Directions:

1. Combine powdered peanut butter, chia seeds, soymilk, salt, syrup, banana, and oats in a medium-sized jar. Ensure all ingredients are mixed thoroughly.
2. Place the jar in the refrigerator and allow the mixture to set overnight.
3. The following day, serve the oats topped with fresh berries or a desired dollop of peanut butter.

Nutritional information

- *Calories*: kcal
- *Total Fat*: g
- *Protein*: g
- *Carbohydrates*: g
- *Sodium*: mg

10. Quark Cucumber Toast

Preparation time: 5 minutes

Cooking time: 5 minutes

Serving: 2

Difficulty level: Easy

Ingredients

- 2 slices of bread
- 4 tbsp (tablespoons) quark
- 4 tbsp (tablespoons) cucumber, finely chopped
- 2 tbsp (tablespoons) fresh cilantro leaves, chopped
- A pinch of sea salt

Directions:

1. Toast the bread slices to your desired level of crispness.
2. Evenly spread quark over each toasted slice.
3. Top with finely chopped cucumber and cilantro.
4. Sprinkle a pinch of sea salt over each slice.
5. Serve immediately and enjoy.

Nutritional information

- *Calories: 141 kcal*
- *Total Fat: 5.1 g*
- *Carbohydrates: 13.8 g*
- *Protein: 7.6 g*
- *Sodium: 299.8 mg*

4.2 Midday Meals: Lunch Options

11. Seafood with Sundried Tomatoes and Pasta

Preparation time: 10 minutes

Cooking time: 10 minutes

Serving: 2

Difficulty level: Easy

Ingredients

- 1/4 cup (60 ml) olive oil
- 4 garlic cloves, minced
- 1 lb (pound) scallops
- 1 lb (pound) shrimp, peeled and deveined
- 1/3 cup sun-dried tomatoes, chopped
- 2 1/2 tsp (teaspoons) lemon zest
- 1/2 tsp (teaspoon) black pepper
- 1 cup (240 ml) water
- 1 lb (pound) whole wheat linguine pasta, cooked
- 1/4 cup fresh parsley, chopped
- A dash of red pepper flakes

Directions:

1. In a skillet, heat the olive oil over medium heat. Once hot, sauté the minced garlic until it becomes fragrant.
2. Add the scallops, shrimp, sun-dried tomatoes, and lemon zest to the skillet.
3. Season the mixture with black pepper and then pour in the water.
4. Cover the skillet with a lid and bring the mixture to a boil.
5. Reduce the heat and let it simmer for approximately 6 minutes.
6. Stir in the cooked linguine pasta and continue cooking for 2 minutes, ensuring the pasta is well-coated with the sauce.
7. Before serving, garnish the dish with freshly chopped parsley and a sprinkle of red pepper flakes.

Nutritional information

- *Calories: 241 kcal*
- *Carbohydrates: 14.6 g*
- *Protein: 22.5 g*
- *Total Fat: 10.3 g*
- *Sodium: 328 mg*

12. Chicken Salad with Oranges

Preparation time: 5 minutes

Cooking time: 15 minutes

Serving: 2

Difficulty level: Medium

Ingredients

- 1/2 cup (120 ml) red wine vinegar
- 2 garlic cloves, minced
- 1 tbsp (tablespoon) olive oil
- 1 tbsp (tablespoon) finely chopped red onion
- 1 tbsp (tablespoon) finely chopped celery
- 1 tbsp (tablespoon) black pepper, or to taste
- 2 boneless chicken breasts
- Leaf lettuce, as desired
- 10 ripe olives
- 2 navel oranges, peeled and segmented

Directions:

1. Combine celery, black pepper, minced garlic, red wine vinegar, chopped onions, and olive oil in a mixing bowl. Mix well.
2. Cover the bowl with plastic wrap and refrigerate the mixture.
3. Preheat a gas grill to medium heat and lightly grease the grill grates with cooking spray.
4. Rub the chicken breasts with the minced garlic, discarding any excess garlic.
5. Place the chicken on the grill until golden brown and fully cooked through.
6. Once cooked, remove the chicken from the grill and let it rest for 5 minutes. After resting, slice the chicken into thin strips.
7. Arrange the orange segments, olives, and leaf lettuce on serving plates.
8. Place the sliced chicken breast on each plate's arranged ingredients.
9. Drizzle the refrigerated dressing over the chicken and serve immediately.

Nutritional information

- *Calories: 237 kcal*
- *Carbohydrates: 12 g*
- *Protein: 27 g*
- *Total Fat: 9 g*
- *Sodium: 199 mg*

13. Crispy Cashew Fish Sticks

Preparation time: 15 minutes

Cooking time: 20 minutes

Serving: 2

Difficulty level: Easy

Ingredients

- 4 skinless haddock fillets (3 oz or 85 grams each)
- 1/2 cup (120 ml) ground unsalted roasted cashews
- 1/4 cup (60 ml) low-sodium bread crumbs
- 1 tsp (teaspoon) fresh thyme, finely chopped
- 1 egg white
- 2 tbsp (tablespoons) water
- 1 tbsp (tablespoon) ground black pepper, or to taste
- Nonstick cooking spray

Directions:

1. Preheat the oven to 400°F (204°C). Line a baking tray with parchment paper.
2. Combine the ground cashews, bread crumbs, and chopped thyme in a small bowl.
3. In a separate small bowl, whisk together the egg white and water.
4. Lightly season each haddock fillet with black pepper. Dip the fillet into the egg-white mixture, ensuring it's fully coated.
5. Dredge the fillet in the cashew-breadcrumb mixture, pressing gently to adhere. Place the coated fillet on the prepared baking tray.
6. Repeat the process for the remaining fillets.
7. Lightly spray the coated fillets with nonstick cooking spray.
8. Bake in the oven for approximately 20 minutes or until golden brown fish sticks are cooked.
9. Serve immediately.

Nutritional information

- *Calories: 282 kcal*
- *Carbohydrates: 14 g*
- *Protein: 21 g*
- *Total Fat: 16 g*
- *Sodium: 249 mg*

14. Cod with Citrus Salad

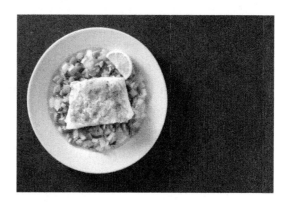

Preparation time: 5 minutes

Cooking time: 10 minutes

Serving: 2

Difficulty level: Easy

Ingredients

- 15 oz (425 grams) cod
- 1 tsp (teaspoon) olive oil
- 1/2 cup (360 ml) spinach, washed and drained
- 1/2 cups (360 ml) kohlrabi, chopped
- 1 cup (240 ml) celery, chopped
- 1/2 cups (360 ml) carrot, julienned
- 2 tbsp (tablespoons) fresh basil, chopped
- 1 tbsp (tablespoon) fresh parsley, chopped
- 3/4 cup (180 ml) red bell pepper, diced
- 1 tbsp (tablespoon) garlic, minced
- Juice of 1 lemon
- Juice of 1 lime
- Juice of 1 orange
- 1 grapefruit, segmented
- 1 orange, segmented
- 1 tbsp (tablespoon) black pepper, or to taste

Directions:

1. Preheat the grill and lightly grease it with cooking spray.

2. Place the cod on the grill and brush it with olive oil. Grill for approximately 10 minutes or until the fish is cooked through. Once done, set it aside.

3. In a large mixing bowl, combine spinach, kohlrabi, celery, carrot, basil, parsley, red bell pepper, garlic, and black pepper. Toss the ingredients gently to mix.

4. Divide the salad between two plates and place a piece of grilled cod on each.

5. Garnish the cod with grapefruit and orange segments.

6. Drizzle the combined lemon, lime, and orange juices over the top and serve immediately.

Nutritional information

- *Calories: 412 kcal*
- *Carbohydrates: 50 g*
- *Protein: 26 g*
- *Total Fat: 12 g*
- *Sodium: 236 mg*

15. Jerk Seasoned Meat Loaves

Preparation time: 5 minutes

Cooking time: 50 minutes

Serving: 2

Difficulty level: Medium

Ingredients

- 2 large eggs, lightly beaten
- 1 medium onion, finely chopped
- 1/2 cup (120 ml) dry bread crumbs
- 2 tbsp (tablespoons) green pepper, finely chopped
- 1 tbsp (tablespoon) Caribbean jerk seasoning
- 2 garlic cloves, minced
- 2 tsp (teaspoons) garlic powder
- 2 tsp (teaspoons) dried cilantro flakes
- 1 tsp (teaspoon) dried basil
- 3 lb (pounds) ground beef

For the Glaze:

- 1/2 cup (120 ml) packed brown sugar
- 2 tbsp (tablespoons) peach nectar or juice
- 2 tbsp (tablespoons) ketchup
- 2 tsp (teaspoons) barbecue sauce
- 1 tbsp (tablespoon) garlic powder
- 1 tbsp (tablespoon) pepper

Directions:

1. Preheat the oven to 350°F (175°C).

2. In a large mixing bowl, combine the first nine ingredients. Gently but thoroughly mix in the ground beef.

3. Transfer the mixture into two ungreased 9-by-5-inch loaf pans.

4. Prepare the glaze in a separate bowl by combining all the ingredients. Spread this glaze evenly over the two meat loaves.

5. Bake in the oven for 40 to 50 minutes or until an internal thermometer reads 160°F (71°C).

6. Allow the meat loaves to rest for 10 minutes before slicing and serving.

Nutritional information

- *Calories: 283 kcal*
- *Total Fat: 14 g*
- *Saturated Fat: 5 g*
- *Protein: 22 g*
- *Cholesterol: 101 mg*
- *Sodium: 223 mg*

16. Grilled Pork Fajitas

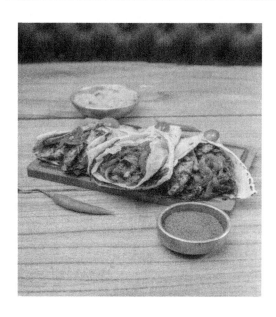

Preparation time: 10 minutes

Cooking time: 5 minutes

Serving: 2

Difficulty level: Hard

Ingredients

- 1 tsp (teaspoon) cumin
- 1/2 tsp (teaspoon) oregano
- 1/2 tsp (teaspoon) paprika
- 1/4 tsp (teaspoon) coriander
- 1/4 tsp (teaspoon) garlic powder
- 1/2 lb (pound) pork tenderloin, sliced
- 1 onion, thinly sliced
- 2 flour tortillas
- 1/2 cup (120 ml) cheddar cheese, shredded
- 2 medium tomatoes, sliced
- 2 cups (480 ml) lettuce, shredded
- 1 cup (240 ml) salsa

Directions:

1. Preheat the broiler to 400°F (204°C).
2. Combine cumin, oregano, coriander, paprika, and garlic powder in a mixing bowl. Mix well.
3. Coat the sliced pork tenderloin evenly with the spice mixture.
4. Place the seasoned pork slices in a grill basket and broil for 5 minutes, turning occasionally to ensure even cooking.
5. Lay out the flour tortillas and evenly distribute the grilled pork and sliced onions between them.
6. Sprinkle shredded cheddar cheese over the pork and onions.
7. Top with tomato slices, shredded lettuce, and a generous spoonful of salsa.
8. Fold the tortillas into a cone wrap shape.

9. Serve immediately, accompanied by additional salsa if desired.

Nutritional information

- *Calories: 180 kcal*
- *Total Fat: 3 g (grams)*
- *Carbohydrates: 29 g (grams)*
- *Protein: 17 g (grams)*
- *Sodium: 382 mg (milligrams)*

! Grilled pork, particularly if the cuts are not lean, can be high in saturated fats, which are known to contribute to heart disease. It is recommended to use lean cuts of pork or substitute with grilled chicken or fish, which are lower in saturated fat and better for maintaining heart health.

17. Pasta Creole Style

Preparation time: 10 minutes

Cooking time: 30 minutes

Serving: 2

Difficulty level: Medium

Ingredients

- 16 oz (ounces) whole wheat pasta
- 1 jar (28 oz or 793 grams) low-sodium pasta sauce
- 1 tsp (teaspoon) Cajun seasoning
- 2 bell peppers, sliced
- 2 medium onions, sliced
- 1 link turkey smoked sausage, sliced
- 1 tbsp (tablespoon) olive oil

Directions:

1. Cook the pasta per the manufacturer's instructions, omitting salt and oil. Once cooked, drain and set aside.
2. Heat a large pot over medium-high heat for 3 minutes.
3. Add the olive oil, ensuring it coats the bottom and sides of the pot.
4. Add the sliced turkey smoked sausage to the pot and cook for 5 minutes, breaking it apart as it cooks. Season with the Cajun seasoning.
5. Incorporate the sliced onions and bell peppers, cooking for 5 minutes.
6. Pour in the jar of low-sodium pasta sauce and allow the mixture to simmer, covered, for 10 minutes.
7. Stir in the cooked pasta, ensuring it's well combined with the sauce.
8. Remove from heat and serve immediately.

Nutritional information

- *Calories: 309 kcal*
- *Total Carbohydrates: 56.6 g*
- *Protein: 8.6 g*
- *Total Fat: 6.0 g*
- *Sodium: 174 mg*

4.3 Evening Culinary Experiences: Dinner Choices

18. Salmon with Marinade

Preparation time: 1 hour 10 minutes

Cooking time: 10 minutes

Serving: 2

Difficulty level: Medium

Ingredients

- 1 cup pineapple juice
- 2 garlic cloves, minced
- 2 tsp (teaspoons) soy sauce
- 1/2 tsp (teaspoon) ginger, finely grated
- 4 salmon fillets
- 1/2 tsp (teaspoon) sesame oil
- 1 tbsp (tablespoon) black pepper, adjusted to taste
- 2 cups fresh fruit, diced

Directions:

1. Combine the pineapple juice, minced garlic, soy sauce, and grated ginger in a mixing bowl. Stir until well combined.
2. Place the salmon fillets in a baking dish.
3. Pour the pineapple mixture over the salmon fillets, ensuring they are well coated. Refrigerate and allow the salmon to marinate for 1 hour.
4. Preheat the oven to 375°F (190°C).
5. Prepare a baking tray by lining it with aluminum foil. Lightly spray the foil with non-stick cooking spray.
6. Transfer the marinated salmon fillets to the prepared baking tray. Drizzle each fillet with sesame oil, then evenly distribute the diced fresh fruit over the salmon. Season with black pepper.
7. Cover the salmon fillets with aluminum foil, sealing the edges to create a pouch.
8. Bake in the oven for 10 minutes or until the salmon is cooked.
9. Remove from the oven, carefully open the foil pouch, and serve immediately.

Nutritional information

- *Calories: 247 kcal*
- *Total Carbohydrates: 19 g*
- *Protein: 27 g*
- *Total Fat: 7 g*
- *Sodium: 192 mg*

19. Balsamic Roast Chicken

Preparation time: 15 minutes

Cooking time: 25 minutes

Serving: 2

Difficulty level: Easy

Ingredients

- 1 lb (pound) chicken
- 1 tbsp (tablespoon) rosemary, finely chopped
- 2 garlic cloves, minced
- 2 tbsp (tablespoon) olive oil
- 1/8 tsp (teaspoon) black pepper, freshly ground
- 4 sprigs fresh rosemary
- 1 cup balsamic vinegar
- 1 tsp (teaspoon) brown sugar

Directions:

1. Preheat the oven to 350°F (175°C).
2. In a mixing bowl, combine the minced garlic and finely chopped rosemary.
3. Rub the chicken with olive oil, ensuring it's well coated. Then, evenly spread the garlic and rosemary mixture over the chicken. Season with freshly ground black pepper. Place the fresh rosemary sprigs inside the chicken cavity.
4. Transfer the chicken to a roasting pan and roast in the preheated oven for 25 minutes or until fully cooked.
5. Once roasted, transfer the chicken to a serving platter.
6. Combine the balsamic vinegar and brown sugar in a saucepan over medium heat. Cook, stirring continuously, until the sugar is completely dissolved.
7. Drizzle the balsamic reduction over the roasted chicken and garnish with additional fresh rosemary sprigs.
8. Serve immediately.

Nutritional information

- *Calories: 301 kcal*
- *Total Carbohydrates: 3 g*
- *Protein: 43 g*
- *Total Fat: 13 g*
- *Sodium: 131 mg*

20. All Spice-Crusted Roasted Salmon

Preparation time: 10 minutes

Cooking time: 20 minutes

Serving: 2

Difficulty level: Medium

Ingredients

- Cooking spray (as needed for coating)
- 1/2 tsp (teaspoon) allspice
- 1/4 tsp (teaspoon) dried basil
- Zest and juice of 1/2 lemon
- 1/4 tsp (teaspoon) dried Italian seasoning
- 1 lb (pound) salmon fillet

Directions:

1. Preheat the oven to 425°F (220°C). Coat a baking sheet with cooking spray.
2. Combine the allspice, dried basil, lemon zest, lemon juice, and Italian seasoning in a small bowl to form a seasoning mixture.

3. Place the salmon fillet on the prepared baking sheet. Evenly spread the seasoning mixture over the salmon.
4. Roast in the preheated oven for 15 to 20 minutes or until the salmon easily flakes with a fork.

Nutritional information

- *Calories: 163 kcal*
- *Total Carbohydrates: 1 g*
- *Protein: 23 g*
- *Total Fat: 7 g*
- *Sodium: 167 mg*

21. Sun-Dried Tomato Turkey Burgers

Preparation time: 15 minutes

Cooking time: 8 minutes

Serving: 2

Difficulty level: Medium

Ingredients

- 1 lb (pound) ground turkey
- 1/2 cup rolled oats
- 1/4 cup sun-dried tomatoes in oil, drained and finely chopped
- 1/4 cup red onion, finely chopped
- 1/4 cup fresh cilantro, finely chopped
- 2 garlic cloves, minced
- 6 whole-wheat hamburger buns
- 1 avocado, pitted and sliced
- 6 lettuce leaves (optional for serving)
- 6 tomato slices (optional for serving)

Directions:

1. Position the oven rack approximately 3 inches from the broiler element and preheat the broiler. Line a rimmed baking sheet with aluminum foil.
2. Combine the ground turkey, rolled oats, sun-dried tomatoes, red onion, cilantro, and minced garlic in a large mixing bowl. Mix until well combined.
3. Shape the mixture into 6 patties, each about 1/2 inch thick.
4. Place the patties on the prepared baking sheet and broil for 3 to 4 minutes on each side until fully cooked and slightly browned.
5. While the patties are broiling, arrange the hamburger buns, avocado slices, lettuce leaves (if using), and tomato slices (if using) on a serving platter.
6. Once the patties are done, allow individuals to assemble their burgers as desired.

Nutritional information

- *Calories: 366 kcal*
- *Total Carbohydrates: 35 g*
- *Protein: 24 g*
- *Total Fat: 15 g*
- *Sodium: 353 mg*

22. Beef and Vegetable Kebabs

Preparation time: 10 minutes

Cooking time: 55 minutes

Serving: 2

Difficulty level: Easy

Ingredients

- 1/2 cup brown rice
- 2 cups water
- 8 oz (ounces) top sirloin, cut into cubes
- 2 tbsp Italian dressing
- 2 green bell peppers, cut into large chunks
- 4 cherry tomatoes
- 2 onions, quartered
- 4 wooden skewers, soaked in water for 20 minutes

Directions:

1. In a saucepan over high heat, combine the water and brown rice. Bring to a boil.
2. Reduce the heat to low, cover, and let the rice simmer for 45 minutes or until tender. Transfer the cooked rice to a serving bowl.
3. In a separate bowl, combine the cubed meat with the Italian dressing. Mix well to ensure the meat is well-coated. Cover with plastic wrap and refrigerate for 20 minutes to marinate.
4. Preheat the grill to medium-high heat and lightly coat with cooking spray. Ensure the cooking rack is positioned about 6 inches from the heat source.
5. Thread the skewers with the ingredients, alternating between green bell pepper chunks, meat cubes, cherry tomatoes, and onion quarters.
6. Place the skewers on the grill and cook for approximately 10 minutes, occasionally turning to ensure even cooking of the vegetables and meat.
7. Serve the kebabs over the cooked brown rice.

Nutritional information

- *Calories: 324 kcal*
- *Total Carbohydrates: 54 g*
- *Protein: 18 g*
- *Total Fat: 4 g*
- *Sodium: 142 mg*

⚠ This recipe includes beef red meat high in saturated fats, especially if the cuts are not lean. For a heart-healthier alternative, consider using skinless chicken or fish. Additionally, ensure that the portion size is appropriate, as excessive consumption of red meat has been linked to increased heart disease risk.

23. Healthy Turkey Chili

Preparation time: 15 minutes

Cooking time: 4-8 hours (4 hours on high or 8 hours on low)

Serving: 2

Difficulty level: Medium

Ingredients

- 2 tbsp extra virgin olive oil
- 1/2 lb (pound) lean ground turkey
- Four 15 oz (ounce) cans of beans: garbanzo, black, kidney, and white kidney, all rinsed and drained
- 1/2 cup red onion, finely chopped
- 3 garlic cloves, minced
- 2 cups fresh tomatoes, chopped
- 2 1/2 cups zucchini, chopped
- 1 tbsp chili powder; 1/4 tsp ground cumin
- 1/2 tsp each of dried parsley, oregano, and basil
- 3 cups low-sodium chicken broth

- 1/8 tsp each of ground black pepper and sea salt
- For garnish: 1/2 cup low-fat cheddar cheese, shredded, and 1/4 cup fresh cilantro, chopped

Directions:

1. In a large sauté pan, heat the olive oil over medium-high heat. Add the ground turkey, onion, and garlic. Cook for 5-6 minutes, stirring constantly to break up the turkey into smaller pieces, until the turkey is browned.
2. Transfer the cooked turkey mixture to a 6-quart slow cooker. Add the beans, tomatoes, zucchini, spices, and chicken broth. Stir to combine.
3. Cover and set the slow cooker to either high for 4 hours or low for 8 hours. Check occasionally, adding water if the mixture appears too dry.
4. Once cooked, ladle the chili into bowls. Garnish with shredded cheddar cheese and chopped cilantro.

Nutritional information

- *Calories: 266 kcal*
- *Total Carbohydrates: 24 g*
- *Protein: 19 g*
- *Total Fat: 11 g*
- *Sodium: 497 mg*

24. Shish Kabob

Preparation time: 15 minutes

Cooking time: 15 minutes

Serving: 2

Difficulty level: Medium

Ingredients

- 24 small onions; 24 cherry tomatoes
- 1/8 tsp ground black pepper; 1/4 tsp salt; Juice of 1 lemon
- 1/2 cup (120 ml) low-sodium chicken broth; 24 mushrooms
- 2 lb (pounds) lean lamb, cut into cubes
- 1/2 tsp dried rosemary; 1 tsp garlic, finely chopped; 1/4 cup (60 ml) red wine; 2 tbsp olive oil

Directions:

1. Combine the red wine, black pepper, salt, olive oil, lemon juice, rosemary, garlic, and chicken broth in a large mixing bowl. Mix well.
2. Add the lamb cubes, mushrooms, tomatoes, and onions to the marinade, ensuring they are well-coated. Refrigerate for 15 minutes to marinate.
3. Preheat the broiler. While heating, thread the marinated lamb, tomatoes, mushrooms, and onions onto skewers.
4. Place the skewers under the broiler and cook for 15 minutes, turning occasionally to ensure even cooking. Once cooked, transfer the skewers to a serving platter. Serve immediately and enjoy.

Nutritional information

- *Calories: 274 kcal*
- *Total Carbohydrates: 16 g*
- *Protein: 26 g; Total Fat: 12 g*
- *Sodium: 20 mg*

4.4 Poultry and Meat: Savory Selections & Marine Delicacies: Fish and Seafood Recipes

25. Chicken with Orzo and Lemon

Preparation time: 10 minutes

Cooking time: 5 to 7 hours

Serving: 2

Difficulty level: Easy

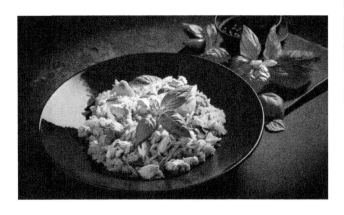

Ingredients

- 3 cups (720 ml) low-sodium chicken broth
- 1 cup (8 oz) uncooked orzo pasta
- 1 lb (pound) boneless, skinless chicken breasts
- 1 lb (pound) carrots, peeled and diced
- 1 small onion, finely diced
- 3 celery stalks, finely diced
- 2 garlic cloves, minced
- 1 tsp dried thyme
- 1 tsp ground turmeric
- 1/2 tsp salt
- 1/2 tsp freshly ground black pepper
- Juice of 1 lemon
- 2 dried bay leaves
- 2 tbsp low-fat feta cheese, crumbled (optional for garnish)

Directions:

1. Combine the chicken broth, orzo pasta, chicken breasts, carrots, onion, celery, garlic, thyme, turmeric, salt, pepper, lemon juice, and bay leaves in a slow cooker. Ensure all ingredients are mixed well.
2. Set the slow cooker to low and cook for 5 to 7 hours.
3. Once cooked, remove and discard the bay leaves. If desired, garnish with crumbled feta cheese before serving.

Nutritional information

- *Calories: 288 kcal*
- *Total Carbohydrates: 30 g*
- *Protein: 34 g*
- *Total Fat: 13 g*
- *Sodium: 427 mg*

26. Mix of Mackerel and Orange

Preparation time: 10 minutes

Cooking time: 20 minutes

Serving: 2

Difficulty level: Medium

Ingredients

- 4 mackerel fillets, skinless and boneless
- 4 spring onions, finely chopped
- 1 tsp (teaspoon) olive oil
- 1-inch piece of ginger, finely grated
- Black pepper, to taste
- Juice and zest of 1 whole orange
- 1 cup (240 ml) low-sodium fish broth

Directions:

1. Season the mackerel fillets with black pepper and lightly brush each fillet with olive oil.
2. Combine the fish broth, orange juice, ginger, orange zest, and chopped spring onions in the Instant Pot.
3. Place a steamer basket inside the Instant Pot and carefully lay the seasoned fillets on the basket.
4. Secure the Instant Pot lid and set it to cook on HIGH pressure for 10 minutes.
5. After the cooking time has elapsed, allow the pressure to release naturally for 10 minutes.
6. Carefully remove the fillets and place them on serving plates. Drizzle the aromatic orange sauce from the pot over the fish fillets.
7. Serve immediately and enjoy.

Nutritional information

- Calories: 200 kcal
- Total Carbohydrates: 19 g (gram)
- Protein: 14 g (gram)
- Total Fat: 4 g (gram)

27. Spicy Chilli Salmon

Preparation time: 10 minutes

Cooking time: 18 minutes

Serving: 2

Difficulty level: Easy

Ingredients

- 4 salmon fillets, boneless with skin on
- 2 tbsp (tablespoons) assorted chili peppers, finely chopped
- Juice of 1 lemon
- 1 lemon, thinly sliced
- 1 cup (240 ml) water
- 1 tbsp (tablespoon) black pepper

Directions:

1. Pour the water into the Instant Pot and insert the steamer basket.

2. Place the salmon fillets on the steamer basket. Season each fillet with black pepper.
3. Drizzle the fresh lemon juice over the salmon fillets.
4. Garnish the salmon with the thinly sliced lemon and chopped chili peppers.
5. Secure the Instant Pot lid and set it to cook on HIGH pressure for 7 minutes.
6. Once the cooking time is complete, allow the pressure to release naturally for 10 minutes.
7. Carefully remove the salmon fillets and lemon slices, placing them on serving plates.
8. Serve immediately and enjoy.

Nutritional information

- *Calories: 281 kcal*
- *Total Carbohydrates: 19 g*
- *Protein: 7 g*
- *Total Fat: 8 g*

28. Salmon Sage Bake

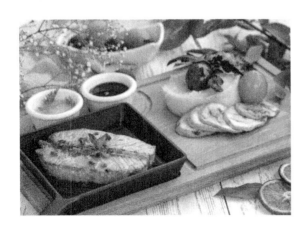

Preparation time: 5 minutes

Cooking time: 15 minutes

Serving: 2

Difficulty level: Easy

Ingredients

- Aluminum foil for lining
- 10 broccoli florets
- 1/4 tsp (teaspoon) ground black pepper
- 1 lime, halved
- 2 salmon fillets (each 4 oz or 113 grams), skin removed
- 2 tbsp (tablespoons) whole-grain mustard
- 1/4 cup (about 4 tbsp) sage, finely chopped

Directions:

1. Preheat the oven to 375°F (190°C). Line a baking sheet with aluminum foil.
2. Arrange the broccoli florets on the baking sheet, seasoning them with ground black pepper.
3. Create two separate beds using five broccoli florets for each salmon fillet. Slice one-half of the lime and place the slices atop the broccoli beds. Position the salmon fillets over the lime slices.
4. Combine the whole-grain mustard and finely chopped sage in a small mixing bowl. Spread this mixture evenly over each salmon fillet.

5. Bake in the preheated oven for approximately 15 minutes or until the salmon appears opaque and can be easily flaked with a fork.

6. Upon serving, squeeze the juice from the reserved lime half over both salmon fillets.

Nutritional information

- *Calories: 171 kcal*
- *Total Carbohydrates: 6 g*
- *Protein: 24 g*
- *Total Fat: 5 g*
- *Sodium: 76 mg*

29. Beef Tenderloin with Balsamic Tomatoes

Preparation time: 5 minutes

Cooking time: 20 minutes

Serving: 2

Difficulty level: Medium

Ingredients

- 1/2 cup (120 ml) balsamic vinegar
- 3/4 cup coarsely chopped, seeded tomato
- 2 tsp (teaspoons) olive oil
- 2 beef tenderloin steaks (each 3-4 oz or 85-113 grams and 3/4-inch thick), trimmed of visible fat
- 1 tsp (teaspoon) fresh thyme (or 1/2 tsp dried thyme)

Directions:

1. In a small saucepan, bring the balsamic vinegar to a boil. Allow it to simmer uncovered until the liquid reduces to approximately 1/4 cup, which should take about 5 minutes.

2. Incorporate the chopped tomatoes into the saucepan and let them simmer for 1-2 minutes. Once done, remove the saucepan from heat.

3. In a large skillet, heat the olive oil over medium-high heat. Once hot, reduce the heat to medium and add the beef tenderloin steaks. Cook the steaks, turning them once, until they reach the desired level of doneness. This should take about 7-9 minutes on each side for medium doneness (160°F or 71°C).

4. Spoon the balsamic tomato mixture over the cooked steaks and sprinkle with thyme.

5. Serve immediately.

Nutritional information

- *Calories: 298 kcal*

- *Total Carbohydrates: 11 g (gram)*
- *Protein: 17 g (gram)*
- *Total Fat: 20 g (gram)*
- *Sodium: 69 mg (milligram)*

30. Flounder with Tomatoes

Preparation time: 10 minutes

Cooking time: 20 minutes

Serving: 2

Difficulty level: Hard

Ingredients

- 4 flounder fillets (each 5-6 oz or 142-170 grams)
- 1 lb (pound) or 16 oz cherry tomatoes
- 4 garlic cloves, thinly sliced
- 2 tbsp (tablespoons) olive oil
- 2 tbsp (tablespoons) lemon juice
- 2 tbsp (tablespoons) fresh basil, cut into ribbons
- 1/2 tsp (teaspoon) kosher salt
- 1/4 tsp (teaspoon) black pepper

Directions:

1. Preheat the oven to 425°F (218°C).
2. Combine the cherry tomatoes, sliced garlic, olive oil, lemon juice, basil ribbons, kosher salt, and black pepper in a baking dish. Mix thoroughly to ensure even seasoning.
3. Place the baking dish in the preheated oven and bake for approximately 5 minutes.
4. After 5 minutes, remove the baking dish from the oven. Carefully arrange the flounder fillets on top of the tomato mixture.
5. Return the dish to the oven and bake for 10 to 15 minutes or until the flounder becomes opaque and easily flakes with a fork. The exact cooking time may vary based on the thickness of the fillets.

Nutritional information

- *Calories: 413 kcal*
- *Total Carbohydrates: 6.9 g*
- *Protein: 39.1 g*
- *Total Fat: 24.5 g*
- *Sodium: 962 mg*

31. Miso-Glazed Tuna

Preparation time: 10 minutes (plus an additional 30 minutes for chilling)

Cooking time: 15 minutes

Serving: 2

Difficulty level: Easy

Ingredients

- Cooking spray
- 1/3 cup white miso
- 1/3 cup sake
- 1/3 cup mirin
- 2 tbsp (tablespoons) brown sugar
- 4 tuna steaks (each 5 oz or 142 grams)

Directions:

1. Preheat the oven to 400°F (204°C). Lightly spray an ovenproof baking dish with cooking spray.
2. Whisk together the white miso, sake, mirin, and brown sugar in a small saucepan set over low heat. Continue whisking until the sugar has fully dissolved, which should take approximately 2 minutes.
3. Transfer the glaze to a medium-sized bowl. Add the tuna steaks, ensuring each piece is well-coated with the glaze. Cover the bowl and refrigerate for a minimum of 30 minutes. Avoid marinating for longer than overnight.
4. Once marinated, remove the tuna steaks from the glaze and arrange them in the prepared baking dish. Any leftover glaze should be discarded.
5. Bake the tuna in the preheated oven for about 12 minutes. The fish should appear opaque and reach an internal temperature of at least 145°F (63°C).
6. The tuna can be served immediately while warm. Alternatively, if you wish to store it for later consumption, allow the fish to cool before transferring it to a freezer-safe container. It can be frozen for up to 2 months. To thaw, place the frozen tuna in the refrigerator overnight. For reheating, microwave a single piece on high for approximately 1 1/2 minutes or reheat in a 350°F (177°C) oven for around 10 minutes.

Nutritional information

- *Calories: 271 kcal*
- *Total Carbohydrates: 23 g*
- *Protein: 37 g*
- *Total Fat: 1 g*
- *Sodium: 959 mg*

32. Chicken Fajitas

Preparation time: 10 minutes

Cooking time: 4 to 6 hours (on low setting)

Serving: 2

Difficulty level: Medium

Ingredients

- 2 1/2 cups salsa
- 2 lb (pounds) boneless, skinless chicken breasts, sliced
- 1 onion, sliced
- 2 bell peppers (seeds removed), sliced
- 2 tbsp (tablespoons) Homemade Fajita Blend

Directions:

1. Evenly spread the salsa at the base of the slow cooker.
2. Add the sliced chicken, onion, bell peppers, and the Homemade Fajita Blend to the slow cooker. Stir the ingredients to ensure they are well-mixed.
3. Set the slow cooker to the low setting and let the mixture cook for 4 to 6 hours.
4. Once cooked, serve the chicken fajitas as desired.

Nutritional information

- *Calories: 201 kcal*
- *Total Carbohydrates: 8 g*
- *Protein: 36 g*
- *Total Fat: 2 g*
- *Sodium: 167 mg*

33. Baked Salmon with Fennel

Preparation time: 10 minutes

Cooking time: 20 minutes

Serving: 2

Difficulty level: Easy

Ingredients

- 1 tbsp (tablespoon) olive oil
- 1 fennel bulb, thinly sliced
- 4 salmon fillets (5 to 6 oz each)
- 1 leek (white part only), thinly sliced
- 1/2 cup vegetable broth (or water as an alternative)
- 1 fresh rosemary sprig
- 1 tsp (teaspoon) salt
- 1/4 tsp (teaspoon) black pepper

Directions:

1. Preheat the oven to 375°F.
2. In a shallow roasting pan, add the olive oil.
3. Add the thinly sliced leek and fennel to the pan, stirring to ensure they are well-coated with the oil.
4. Place the salmon fillets atop the vegetables. Season the fillets with salt and black pepper.
5. Pour the vegetable broth over the salmon and vegetables, then place the rosemary sprig in the pan.
6. Tightly cover the pan with aluminum foil.
7. Transfer the pan to the preheated oven and bake for approximately 20 minutes or until the salmon is thoroughly cooked.
8. Once cooked, remove and discard the rosemary sprig.
9. Serve the salmon and vegetables immediately.

Nutritional information

- *Calories: 408 kcal*

- *Total Carbohydrates: 27.7 g*
- *Protein: 24.4 g*
- *Total Fat: 23.1 g*
- *Sodium: 412 mg*

---

34. Beef Stroganoff

Preparation time: 10 minutes

Cooking time: 25 minutes

Serving: 2

Difficulty level: Easy

Ingredients

- 1/2 cup chopped onion
- 1/2 lb (pound) boneless beef round steak, cut into 3/4-inch thick pieces
- 4 cups pasta noodles
- 1/2 cup fat-free cream of mushroom soup
- 1/2 cup water
- 1/2 tsp (teaspoon) paprika
- 1/2 cup fat-free sour cream, low-fat yogurt, or a plant-based cream alternative.

Directions:

1. In a non-stick frying pan, sauté the onions over medium heat until translucent, stirring for about 5 minutes.
2. Add the beef to the pan and continue to cook until the beef is browned on all sides and tender. Remove from heat and set aside.
3. In a large pot, bring water to a boil. Add the pasta noodles and cook according to the package instructions. Once cooked, drain and set aside.
4. In a separate saucepan, combine the cream of mushroom soup and water. Whisk together and bring to a boil over medium heat, stirring constantly. Once the mixture has thickened slightly, stir in the paprika and sour cream.
5. To serve, place the cooked pasta in bowls, top with the beef and onion mixture, and pour the sauce over the top.
6. Serve immediately while warm.

Nutritional information

- *Calories: 273 kcal*
- *Total Carbohydrates: 37 g*
- *Protein: 20 g*
- *Total Fat: 5 g*
- *Sodium: 193 mg*

⚠ Beef Stroganoff traditionally includes a cream-based sauce, which can be high in saturated fats. Consider using a low-fat yogurt or a plant-based cream alternative to make this dish more heart-friendly. Additionally, opt for lean cuts of beef or replace beef with a leaner protein source.

35. Pork Tenderloin with Fennel and Orange

Preparation time: 10 minutes

Cooking time: 20 minutes

Serving: 2

Difficulty level: Easy

Ingredients

- 2 pork tenderloin fillets
- 2 tbsp (tablespoons) olive oil
- 1 tsp (teaspoon) fennel seeds
- 1 fennel bulb, thinly sliced
- 1 sweet onion, chopped
- 1/2 cup dry white wine
- 12 oz (ounces) chicken broth
- Fennel fronds (from the fennel bulb) for garnish
- 4 orange slices

Directions:

1. Place the pork tenderloin between two sheets of wax paper. Cover with another two sheets. Flatten the pork using a mallet or rolling pin until it's about 1/4 inch thick.
2. In a large skillet, heat the olive oil over medium heat. Add the fennel seeds and cook until fragrant, about 3 minutes. Add the pork and cook for approximately 3 minutes on each side or until fully cooked. Transfer the pork to a plate and cover to keep warm.
3. In the same skillet, sauté the onions and sliced fennel until tender, about 5 minutes. Transfer the vegetables to a bowl and cover to keep warm.
4. Pour the white wine and chicken broth into the skillet. Bring to a boil over high heat and reduce by half. Return the pork to the skillet, cover, and simmer for 5 minutes on low heat.
5. Add the sautéed fennel and onion mixture to the skillet and juice from the orange slices. Cover and cook for an additional 2 minutes.
6. Serve the pork and vegetables on warmed plates, garnished with fennel fronds and orange slices.

Nutritional information

- *Calories: 276 kcal*
- *Total Carbohydrates: 13 g*
- *Protein: 29 g*
- *Total Fat: 12 g*
- *Sodium: 122 mg*

36. Roasted Salmon with Fresh Herbs

Preparation time: 10 minutes

Cooking time: 12-14 minutes

Serving: 2

Difficulty level: Medium

Ingredients

- 2 salmon fillets
- 2 tsp (teaspoons) olive oil
- 1 tbsp (tablespoon) chives, finely chopped
- 1 tbsp (tablespoon) tarragon leaves, finely chopped

Directions:

1. Preheat the oven to 425°F (Fahrenheit). Line a baking sheet with foil.
2. Lightly rub each salmon fillet with olive oil and place them skin side down on the prepared baking sheet.
3. Bake in the preheated oven for approximately 10 minutes. Check the salmon for doneness by flaking it with a fork. If not fully cooked, continue baking for 2-4 minutes or until the fish is cooked through and flakes easily.
4. Using a metal spatula, carefully lift the salmon off the baking sheet, leaving the skin behind, and transfer it to serving plates.
5. Garnish the salmon with the finely chopped chives and tarragon leaves. Serve immediately.

Nutritional information

- *Calories: 244 kcal*
- *Total Carbohydrates: 0.1 g*
- *Protein: 28 g*
- *Total Fat: 14 g*
- *Sodium: 63 mg*

37. Roasted Salmon with Maple-Balsamic Glaze

Preparation time: 10 minutes

Cooking time: 35 minutes

Serving: 2

Difficulty level: Hard

Ingredients

- 1/4 cup maple syrup
- 1 garlic clove, minced
- 1/4 cup balsamic vinegar
- 1 lb salmon fillets
- 1/4 tsp (teaspoon) kosher salt
- 1/8 tsp (teaspoon) black pepper
- 1 tbsp (tablespoon) fresh mint, finely chopped (for garnish)

Directions:

1. Preheat the oven to 450°F (Fahrenheit). Lightly coat a baking pan with cooking spray.
2. Combine the maple syrup, minced garlic, and balsamic vinegar in a small saucepan over low heat. Warm the mixture until it's just heated, then remove from heat. Set aside half of this glaze for serving.
3. Pat the salmon fillets dry and place them skin-side down on the prepared baking pan. Generously brush the salmon with the maple-balsamic glaze.

4. Bake the salmon in the preheated oven for approximately 10 minutes, reapplying the glaze every 5 minutes. Continue baking for 20-25 minutes or until the salmon easily flakes with a fork.

5. Plate the cooked salmon fillets, season with kosher salt and black pepper, and drizzle with the reserved glaze. Garnish with finely chopped fresh mint before serving.

Nutritional information

- *Calories: 257 kcal*
- *Total Carbohydrates: 10 g*
- *Protein: 30 g*
- *Total Fat: 10 g*
- *Sodium: 167 mg*

38. Spicy Beef Kebabs

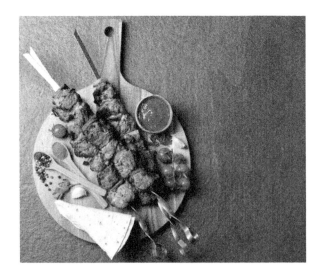

Preparation time: 10 minutes

Cooking time: 10 minutes

Serving: 2

Difficulty level: Medium

Ingredients

- 2 yellow onions, finely minced
- 2 tbsp (tablespoon) fresh lemon juice
- 1 1/2 lb (pounds) lean ground beef
- 1/4 cup bulgur, soaked in water for 30 minutes and then drained
- 1/4 cup pine nuts, finely chopped
- 2 garlic cloves, minced
- 1 tsp (teaspoon) ground cumin
- 1/2 tsp (teaspoon) ground cinnamon
- 1/2 tsp (teaspoon) ground cardamom
- 1/2 tsp (teaspoon) freshly ground black pepper
- 16 wooden skewers soaked in water for 30 minutes

Directions:

1. Combine onions, lemon juice, ground beef, drained bulgur, pine nuts, garlic, and spices in a large mixing bowl. Mix until well combined.

2. Take a portion of the meat mixture and shape it into a sausage-like form. Thread each portion onto a soaked wooden skewer. If the mixture is too crumbly, add 1 tbsp at a time until it binds together. Place the skewered kebabs in the refrigerator until ready to grill.

3. Preheat the grill to 350°F, positioning the grill rack approximately 6 inches from the heat source.

4. Grill the kebabs for about 5 minutes on each side or until they are cooked

through and have a nice char on the outside.

Nutritional information

- *Calories: 219 kcal*
- *Total Carbohydrates: 3 g*
- *Protein: 23 g*
- *Total Fat: 12 g*
- *Sodium: 53 mg*

⚠ Spicy beef kebabs may contain high sodium levels, particularly if pre-made spice mixes are used. High sodium intake is a risk factor for hypertension, a leading cause of heart disease. Use fresh herbs and spices to flavor the kebabs instead of salt-heavy mixes, and choose lean cuts of beef or a heart-healthier protein like chicken or fish.

39. Curried Pork Tenderloin in Apple Cider

Preparation time: 10 minutes

Cooking time: 26 minutes

Serving: 2

Difficulty level: Easy

Ingredients

- 16 oz (ounces) pork tenderloin, sectioned into 6 pieces
- 1 1/2 tbsp (tablespoon) curry powder
- 1 tbsp (tablespoon) extra-virgin olive oil
- 2 medium-sized onions, finely chopped
- 2 cups organic, unsweetened apple cider
- 1 tart apple, peeled and segmented into chunks

Directions:

1. In a mixing bowl, thoroughly coat the pork pieces with curry powder. Set aside for marination.
2. In a pot, warm the olive oil over medium heat.
3. Add the chopped onions, sautéing until they release their aroma, approximately 1 minute.
4. Introduce the seasoned pork tenderloin to the pot. Cook until the pork adopts a light golden hue, which should take around 5 minutes.
5. Pour in the apple cider and incorporate the apple chunks.
6. Secure the pot with its lid and elevate the heat to achieve a boil.
7. Once boiling, reduce the heat and let the mixture simmer for 20 minutes.

Nutritional information

- *Calories: 244 kcal*
- *Total Carbohydrates: 18 g*
- *Protein: 24 g*

- *Total Fat: 8 g*
- *Sodium: 70 mg*

⚠ Pork tenderloin is a leaner cut of pork, which is a positive choice for heart health. However, it is important to consider the cooking method and the ingredients used in the marinade or sauce. Avoid using high-sodium ingredients and use natural spices and herbs to enhance flavor without adding excess salt.

40. Seafood Tomato Stew

Preparation time: 10 minutes

Cooking time: 11 minutes

Serving: 2

Difficulty level: Medium

Ingredients

- 2 tbsp (tablespoon) olive oil
- 8 oz (ounces) cod, with pin bones meticulously removed and diced
- 8 oz (ounces) shrimp, both peeled and deveined
- 1 can (14 oz) tomato sauce
- 1 medium-sized onion, finely chopped
- 1 garlic clove, minced
- 1/2 cup dry white wine
- 1 tbsp (tablespoon) Italian seasoning blend
- 1/2 tsp (teaspoon) sea salt
- A pinch of red pepper flakes

Directions:

1. Heat the olive oil over medium-high heat in a skillet suitable for stews until it exhibits a shimmering appearance.
2. Incorporate the chopped onion, sautéing for approximately 3 minutes until translucent.
3. Introduce the minced garlic, allowing it to cook for about 30 seconds, ensuring it doesn't brown.
4. Pour in the white wine, stirring continuously for around 1 minute to allow the alcohol to evaporate.
5. Blend in the tomato sauce and bring the mixture to a gentle simmer.
6. Introduce the diced cod, shrimp, Italian seasoning, sea salt, and red pepper flakes to the skillet.
7. Allow the mixture to simmer roughly 5 minutes or until the seafood becomes opaque and fully cooked.
8. Serve the stew immediately, preferably with crusty bread or overcooked rice.

Nutritional information

- *Calories: 236 kcal*
- *Total Carbohydrates: 9.8 g*
- *Protein: 25.7 g*
- *Total Fat: 10.4 g*
- *Sodium: 713 mg*

41. Cod Cauliflower Chowder

Preparation time: 15 minutes

Cooking time: 40minutes

Serving: 2

Difficulty level: Easy

Ingredients

- 2 tbsp (tablespoon) olive oil
- 1 1/2 lb (pounds) cod, cut into bite-sized pieces
- 1 leek, cleaned and thinly sliced
- 1 medium-sized cauliflower head, chopped into small florets
- 2 pints cherry tomatoes
- 4 garlic cloves, thinly sliced
- 1 tsp (teaspoon) kosher salt
- 1/4 tsp (teaspoon) freshly ground black pepper
- 2 cups no-salt-added vegetable stock
- 1/4 cup green olives, pitted and finely chopped
- 1/4 cup fresh parsley, minced

Directions:

1. Warm the olive oil over medium heat in a large Dutch oven or pot.
2. Introduce the sliced leek and sauté until it achieves a light golden hue, approximately 5 minutes.
3. Incorporate the sliced garlic, allowing it to cook for 30 seconds without browning.
4. Add the chopped cauliflower, seasoning with salt and black pepper, and continue sautéing for 2 to 3 minutes.

5. Introduce the cherry tomatoes and vegetable stock, then increase the heat to high, bringing the mixture to a boil.
6. Once boiling, reduce the heat to low, allowing the mixture to simmer for roughly 10 minutes.
7. Blend in the chopped olives. Subsequently, nestle the cod pieces into the mixture, ensuring they are submerged. Cover the pot and let it simmer for 20 minutes or until the cod becomes opaque and easily flakes when tested with a fork.
8. Stir gently in the minced parsley, ensuring it does not break the fish.
9. Serve the chowder immediately, accompanied by crusty bread if desired.

Nutritional information

- *Calories: 427 kcal*
- *Total Carbohydrates: 13.7 g*
- *Protein: 51.2 g*
- *Total Fat: 18.1 g*
- *Sodium: 676 mg*

42. Steamed Salmon Teriyaki

Preparation time: 15 minutes

Cooking time: 15 minutes

Serving: 2

Difficulty level: Hard

Ingredients

- 3 green onions, finely chopped
- 2 packets of Stevia
- 1 tbsp (tablespoon) freshly grated ginger
- 1 garlic clove, minced
- 2 tsp (teaspoon) sesame seeds
- 1 tbsp (tablespoon) sesame oil
- 1/4 cup mirin
- 2 tbsp (tablespoon) low-sodium soy sauce
- 1/2 lb (pound) salmon fillet

Directions:

1. Position a large saucepan over medium-high heat. Insert a trivet into the saucepan and fill it halfway with water. Secure the lid and bring the water to a boil.
2. Combine Stevia, ginger, garlic, sesame oil, mirin, and soy sauce in a heat-resistant dish that can comfortably fit inside the saucepan. Introduce the salmon to this mixture, ensuring it's thoroughly coated.
3. Sprinkle the salmon with sesame seeds and the finely chopped green onions. Tightly cover the dish with aluminum foil.
4. Position the dish atop the trivet within the saucepan. Seal the saucepan with its lid and allow the salmon to steam for approximately 15 minutes.
5. Once cooked, let the salmon sit in the pan for 5 minutes.
6. Serve the salmon immediately, drizzling any remaining sauce over the top.

Nutritional information

- *Calories: 242.7 kcal*
- *Total Carbohydrates: 1.2 g*
- *Protein: 35.4 g*
- *Total Fat: 10.7 g*
- *Sodium: 285 mg*

43. Salmon, Spinach, and Lasagna

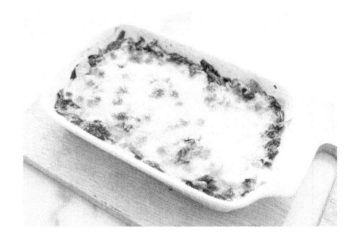

Preparation time: 30 minutes

Cooking time: 1 hour

Serving: 2

Difficulty level: Easy

Ingredients

- 1 1/2 cups white wine
- 2 garlic cloves, lightly crushed
- 4 tbsp (tablespoon) fresh dill
- 1/4 tsp (teaspoon) salt
- 1 tsp (teaspoon) freshly ground black pepper
- 1 lb (pound) salmon fillet
- 16 oz (ounce) whole-wheat lasagna noodles, cooked to al dente
- 1 cup baby spinach
- 1 cup nonfat or low-fat plain Greek yogurt
- 2 cups part-skim mozzarella cheese, shredded

Directions:

1. Preheat the oven to 350°F.
2. Combine white wine, garlic, dill, salt, and pepper in a shallow saucepan. Heat to a gentle simmer. Introduce the salmon fillet and poach until fully cooked, turning it once. Remove from heat, cool, and flake the salmon into bite-sized pieces. Place in the refrigerator for 15 minutes.
3. Lightly oil a 9-by-13-inch baking dish. Begin layering the dish by placing 1/3 of the lasagna noodles at the base, followed by equal portions of spinach, salmon, Greek yogurt, and mozzarella cheese. Repeat this layering process twice, ensuring the final layer is topped with mozzarella cheese.
4. Transfer the baking dish to the oven and bake for approximately 30 to 35 minutes, or until the cheese has melted and turned a golden brown hue.
5. Once baked, allow the lasagna to cool for 5 to 10 minutes before serving.

Nutritional information

- *Calories: 385 kcal*
- *Total Carbohydrates: 46 g*
- *Protein: 29 g*
- *Total Fat: 9 g*
- *Sodium: 310 mg*

4.5 Comfort in a Bowl: Dressings and Soups

44. Herbed Smashed Potatoes with Garlic

Preparation time: 20 minutes

Cooking time: 5 to 6 hours

Serving: 2

Difficulty level: Medium

Ingredients

- 3 1/2 lb (pounds) red or creamer potatoes, thoroughly rinsed
- 2 onions, finely minced
- 12 garlic cloves, peeled and thinly sliced
- 1/2 cup roasted vegetable broth
- 3 tbsp (tablespoon) olive oil
- 1 tsp (teaspoon) dried thyme leaves
- 1 tsp (teaspoon) dried dill leaves
- 1/2 tsp (teaspoon) salt
- 1/3 cup grated Parmesan cheese

Directions:

1. In a 6-quart slow cooker, combine the potatoes, onions, garlic, vegetable broth, olive oil, thyme, dill, and salt. Ensure all ingredients are mixed well.
2. Cover the slow cooker and set it to cook on low. Allow the mixture to cook for 5 to 6 hours or until the potatoes have become tender.
3. Once cooked, use a potato masher to smash the potatoes within the slow cooker gently. Aim to leave some pieces slightly chunky for texture.
4. Stir in the grated Parmesan cheese until well combined.
5. Serve the herbed smashed potatoes while hot.

Nutritional information

- *Calories: 321 kcal*
- *Total Carbohydrates: 48 g*
- *Protein: 10 g(gram)*
- *Total Fat: 10 g*
- *Sodium: 439 mg*

45. Celery Sticks with Chipotle Aioli Dip

Preparation time: 20 minutes

Cooking time: 1 hour

Serving: 2

Difficulty level: Hard

Ingredients

- 3/4 cup raw cashews
- 1/2 cup almond milk
- 2 tbsp (tablespoon) lemon juice
- 1/2 tsp (teaspoon) coconut aminos
- 1 packet stevia
- 2 whole chipotle peppers in adobo sauce, plus 1 tbsp (tablespoon) reserved adobo sauce
- Pinch of smoked paprika
- 6 celery stalks, each cut into 3-inch lengths
- Boiling water (for soaking)

Directions:

1. In a mixing bowl, add the cashews and cover them with boiling water. Allow them to soak for 1 hour, then drain thoroughly.
2. Transfer the drained cashews to a blender. Add almond milk, lemon juice, coconut aminos, stevia, chipotle peppers, reserved adobo sauce, and smoked paprika.
3. Blend the mixture until it achieves a smooth and creamy consistency.
4. Transfer the aioli dip to a serving bowl and serve alongside the prepared celery sticks.

Nutritional information

- *Calories: 52 kcal*
- *Total Carbohydrates: 5.0 g*
- *Protein: 1.7 g*
- *Total Fat: 3.3 g*
- *Sodium: 22mg*

46. Appetizing Cucumber Salad

Preparation time: 30 minutes

Cooking time: 20 minutes (No cooking required)

Serving: 2

Difficulty level: Easy

Ingredients

- 2 cucumbers, peeled
- 1/2 cup sour cream
- 2 tbsp (tablespoon) low-fat, low-sodium mayonnaise
- 1 tsp (teaspoon) mustard
- 1 tbsp (tablespoon) fresh lemon juice
- 1 garlic clove, minced
- 1/3 cup fresh dill leaves, coarsely chopped
- 1/2 tsp (teaspoon) black pepper

Directions:

1. Cut each cucumber into three equal lengths. Then, slice each lengthwise into quarters or smaller to produce cucumber sticks. Allow the cucumber sticks to drain in a colander.
2. In a medium-sized bowl, whisk together sour cream, mayonnaise, mustard, lemon juice, minced garlic, chopped dill, and black pepper until well combined.
3. Add the drained cucumber sticks to the dressing, ensuring they are well coated.

4. Serve immediately.

Nutritional information

- *Calories: 37.9 kcal*
- *Total Carbohydrates: 3.3 g*
- *Protein: 1 g*
- *Total Fat: 2.3 g*
- *Sodium: 24 mg*

47. Celery and Chili Peppers Stir Fry

Preparation time: 10 minutes

Cooking time: 5 minutes

Serving: 2

Difficulty level: Easy

Ingredients

- 2 tbsp (tablespoon) olive oil
- 3 dried chili peppers, crushed
- 4 cups julienned celery
- 2 tbsp (tablespoon) coconut aminos

Directions:

1. In a skillet or pan, heat the olive oil over medium-high heat. Once hot, add the crushed chili peppers and sauté for 2 minutes, stirring frequently.
2. Incorporate the julienned celery and coconut aminos into the pan. Continue to stir and cook for an additional 3 minutes.

3. Transfer the stir fry to serving plates and serve immediately, preferably as a side dish.

Nutritional information

- Calories: 42 kcal
- Total Carbohydrates: 7.2 g
- Protein: 1.5 g
- Total Fat: 2 g

48. Roasted Brussels Sprouts

Preparation time: 5 minutes

Cooking time: 20 minutes

Serving: 2

Difficulty level: Easy

Ingredients

- 1 1/2 lbs (pounds) Brussels sprouts, trimmed and halved
- 2 tbsp (tablespoon) olive oil
- 1/4 tsp (teaspoon) salt
- 1/2 tsp (teaspoon) freshly ground black pepper

Directions:

1. Preheat the oven to 400°F (degrees Fahrenheit).
2. Combine the Brussels sprouts with olive oil in a large mixing bowl, ensuring they are evenly coated.

3. Transfer the Brussels sprouts to a large baking sheet, positioning them to cut side down.
4. Season the Brussels sprouts with salt and pepper.
5. Roast in the oven for 20 to 30 minutes or until the Brussels sprouts are lightly charred and crispy outside with a toasted bottom. Note: The outer leaves may darken significantly.
6. Serve immediately.

Nutritional information

- Calories: 106 kcal
- Total Carbohydrates: 11 g
- Protein: 4 g
- Total Fat: 7 g

49. Sautéed Garlic Mushrooms

Preparation time: 10 minutes

Cooking time: 10 minutes

Serving: 2

Difficulty level: Easy

Ingredients

- 1 tbsp (tablespoon) olive oil
- 3 garlic cloves, minced
- 16 oz (ounces) fresh brown mushrooms, sliced
- 7 oz (ounces) fresh shiitake mushrooms, sliced
- 1/2 tsp (teaspoon) salt
- 1/2 tsp (teaspoon) pepper (adjust to taste)

Directions:

1. Preheat a nonstick saucepan over medium-high heat for 1 minute.
2. Add the olive oil and heat for an additional 2 minutes.
3. Incorporate the minced garlic and sauté for 1 minute.
4. Introduce the sliced mushrooms, salt, and pepper. Stir continuously until the mushrooms are soft and tender, approximately 5 minutes.
5. Remove from heat, cover the saucepan, and allow the mushrooms to rest for 5 minutes.
6. Serve immediately.

Nutritional information

- Calories: 44 kcal
- Total Carbohydrates: 2 g
- Protein: 2.2 g
- Total Fat: 3.5 g

50. Pesto Stuffed Mushrooms

Preparation time: 10 minutes

Cooking time: 25 minutes

Serving: 2

Difficulty level: Hard

Ingredients

- 6 large cremini mushrooms
- 6 slices of bacon
- 2 tbsp (tablespoon) basil pesto
- 5 tbsp (tablespoon) low-fat cream cheese, softened

Directions:

1. Preheat the oven to 375°F (Fahrenheit) and line a baking sheet with foil.
2. Thoroughly combine the basil pesto and softened cream cheese in a small mixing bowl.
3. Detach the stems from the mushrooms and discard them. Generously fill each mushroom cap with the pesto-cream cheese mixture.
4. Take a slice of bacon and wrap it securely around a stuffed mushroom. Ensure the entire mushroom is covered. Repeat this step for the remaining mushrooms.
5. Arrange the bacon-wrapped mushrooms on the prepared baking sheet. Bake in the preheated oven for approximately 25 minutes or until the bacon is crispy.
6. Allow the mushrooms to cool slightly before serving.

Nutritional information

- Calories: 137.8 kcal
- Total Carbohydrates: 2 g
- Protein: 5 g
- Total Fat: 12.2 g
- Sodium: 168 mg

---

51. Spicy Refried Beans

Preparation time: 10 minutes

Cooking time: 9 hours

Serving: 2

Difficulty level: Easy

Ingredients

- 4 cups dried pinto beans, rinsed and drained
- 2 onions, finely minced
- 4 garlic cloves, minced
- 1 jalapeño pepper, minced (seeds removed for less heat, if preferred)
- 1 tsp (teaspoon) dried oregano leaves
- 1 tsp (teaspoon) salt
- 9 cups Roasted Vegetable Broth
- 1/3 cup olive oil

Directions:

1. In a 6-quart slow cooker, combine the pinto beans, onions, garlic, jalapeño pepper, oregano, salt, and vegetable broth. Ensure all ingredients are mixed well.
2. Cover the slow cooker and set it to cook on low for approximately 8 hours. The beans should absorb most of the broth and become tender by the end of this period.
3. Uncover the slow cooker and incorporate the olive oil. Using a potato masher, mash the beans directly in the slow cooker until they reach the desired consistency.
4. Continue to cook the beans on low for an additional 30 to 40 minutes. If a thicker consistency is desired, remove the cover and cook on high for an extra 40 to 50 minutes, stirring occasionally to prevent sticking.
5. Once the beans have achieved the desired consistency, serve them warm.

Nutritional information

- Calories: 444 kcal
- Total Carbohydrates: 66 g
- Total Fat: 10 g
- Protein: 21 g
- Sodium: 469 mg

52. Orange Herbed Cauliflower

Preparation time: 20 minutes

Cooking time: 4 hours

Serving: 2

Difficulty level: Medium

Ingredients

- 2 heads cauliflower, thoroughly rinsed and segmented into florets
- 2 onions, finely chopped
- 1/2 cup (120 ml) orange juice
- 1 tsp (teaspoon) freshly grated orange zest
- 1 tsp (teaspoon) dried thyme leaves
- 1/2 tsp (teaspoon) dried basil leaves
- 1/2 tsp (teaspoon) salt

Directions:

1. In a 6-quart slow cooker, combine the cauliflower florets and chopped onions.
2. Pour the orange juice over the cauliflower and onions, ensuring even distribution.
3. Sprinkle the mixture with orange zest, thyme, basil, and salt, ensuring even coverage.
4. Cover the slow cooker and set it to cook on low for approximately 4 hours. The cauliflower should be tender and easily pierced with a fork by the end of the cooking time.
5. Serve warm as a flavorful side dish.

Nutritional information

- *Calories: 75 kcal*
- *Total Carbohydrates: 16 g*
- *Total Fat: 0 g*
- *Saturated Fat: 0 g*

- *Protein: 5 g*
- *Sodium: 212 mg*

53. Mushroom Risotto

Preparation time: 20 minutes

Cooking time: 3.5 to 4.5 hours

Serving: 2

Difficulty level: Easy

Ingredients

- 8 oz (ounces) button mushrooms, thinly sliced
- 8 oz (ounces) cremini mushrooms, thinly sliced
- 8 oz (ounces) shiitake mushrooms, stems discarded and thinly sliced
- 2 onions, finely chopped
- 5 garlic cloves, minced
- 2 cups (16 oz) short-grain brown rice
- 1 tsp (teaspoon) dried marjoram leaves
- 6 cups (48 oz) Roasted Vegetable Broth
- 3 tbsp (tablespoons) unsalted butter
- 1/2 cup (4 oz) grated Parmesan cheese

Directions:

1. In a 6-quart slow cooker, combine the three types of mushrooms, onions, garlic, rice, marjoram, and vegetable broth.
2. Cover the slow cooker and set it to cook on low for approximately 3 to 4 hours. The rice should be tender by the end of the cooking time.
3. Stir in the unsalted butter and grated Parmesan cheese, ensuring even distribution.
4. Cover the slow cooker once more and let the risotto cook on low for an additional 20 minutes.
5. Serve the risotto warm, garnishing with additional Parmesan cheese if desired.

Nutritional information

- *Calories: 331 kcal*
- *Total Carbohydrates: 51 g*
- *Total Fat: 10 g*
- *Protein: 11 g*
- *Sodium: 368 mg*

54. Turkey and Beans Soup

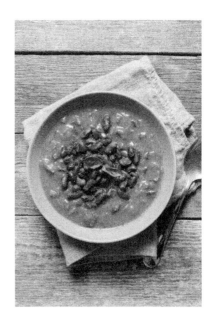

Preparation time: 20 minutes

Cooking time: 30 minutes

Serving: 2

Difficulty level: Medium

- Calories: 242 kcal;
- Total Carbohydrates: 30 g
- Total Fat: 2 g; Protein: 26 g
- Sodium: 204 mg

Ingredients

- 1 lb (pound) ground turkey breast
- 2 medium onions, finely chopped
- 2 celery stalks, finely chopped
- 1 garlic clove, minced
- 1/4 cup (2 oz) ketchup
- 1 can (14.5 oz) unsalted diced tomatoes
- 3 low-sodium chicken bouillon cubes
- 7 cups (56 oz) water
- 1 1/2 tsp (teaspoon) dried basil leaves
- 1/4 tsp (teaspoon) ground black pepper
- 2 cups (16 oz) shredded cabbage
- 1 can (15 oz) unsalted cannellini beans, thoroughly rinsed and drained

Directions:

1. In a large pot over medium heat, sauté the celery, garlic, onion, and ground turkey. Cook until the vegetables are softened, and the turkey is fully cooked.

2. Add the ketchup, diced tomatoes, chicken bouillon cubes, water, dried basil, and ground black pepper to the pot. Stir to combine.

3. Add the shredded cabbage and cannellini beans to the pot and mix well.

4. Cover the pot and let the soup simmer for approximately 30 minutes, stirring occasionally.

5. Once cooked, serve the soup hot, garnishing it with fresh herbs if desired.

4.6 Plant-Based Choices: Salads, Beans, Legumes, and Grains

55. Asparagus Pasta

Preparation time: 20 minutes

Cooking time: 25 minutes

Serving: 2

Difficulty level: Easy

Ingredients

- 1 1/2 lb (pound) fresh asparagus, trimmed and cut into 1-inch pieces
- 8 oz (ounce) angel hair pasta
- 1 tbsp (tablespoon) olive oil
- 1/4 cup (2 oz) chicken broth
- 1/2 tsp (teaspoon) crushed red pepper
- 1/2 lb (pound) fresh mushrooms, sliced
- 1/2 cup (4 oz) grated Parmesan cheese

Directions:

1. Cook the angel hair pasta according to the package instructions until al dente. Drain and set aside.
2. In a large, non-stick skillet, heat the olive oil over medium heat. Add the asparagus pieces and sauté for about 3 minutes.
3. Pour in the chicken broth and add the sliced mushrooms to the skillet. Continue to cook for an additional 3 minutes or until the mushrooms are tender and the asparagus is cooked but still crisp.
4. Transfer the drained pasta to a serving dish. Gently toss the pasta with the asparagus and mushroom mixture.
5. Sprinkle the dish with grated Parmesan cheese and crushed red pepper. Toss again to combine and serve immediately.

Nutritional information

- *Calories: 281 kcal*
- *Total Carbohydrates: 39.4 g*
- *Total Fat: 8.4 g*
- *Protein: 15.5 g*

56. Black Bean Spread with Maple Syrup

Preparation time: 10 minutes

Cooking time: None required

Serving: 2

Difficulty level: Medium

Ingredients

- 4 cups (32 oz) cooked black beans or 2 (15 oz) cans, drained and rinsed
- 6 garlic cloves, peeled and smashed
- Zest of 1 lemon
- Juice of 2 lemons
- 1 tbsp (tablespoon) maple syrup
- 3 tsp (teaspoons) fresh mint, chopped
- Salt, to taste
- 1 cup (8 oz) water, more if needed for consistency

Directions:

1. In a blender, combine the black beans, garlic, lemon zest, lemon juice, chopped mint, maple syrup, salt, and water.
2. Blend until the mixture is smooth and creamy. If the spread is too thick, add more water in small increments until the desired consistency is achieved.
3. Transfer the spread to a serving dish and serve as desired.

Nutritional information

- *Calories: 52 kcal*
- *Total Fat: 0.2 g*
- *Sodium: 2 mg*
- *Total Carbohydrates: 11 g*
- *Protein: 2.4 g*

57. Grilled Vegetable and Pineapple Salad

Preparation time: 10 minutes

Cooking time: None required

Serving: 2

Difficulty level: Easy

Ingredients

- Vegetables from 1/2 batch of Grilled Vegetable Kabobs, removed from skewers
- 2 cups (16 oz) cooked red beans, or 1 (15 oz) can, drained and rinsed
- 1/2 cup fresh dill, finely chopped
- 2 tbsp (tablespoon) maple syrup
- 1/2 tsp (teaspoon) cayenne pepper
- 1/2 pineapple, peeled and diced
- 1 tbsp toasted peanuts
- 1 tbsp salt

Directions:

1. In a large bowl, combine all the ingredients.
2. Toss the mixture until well combined.
3. Chill the salad in the refrigerator for at least 1 hour before serving.

Nutritional information

- *Calories: 129 kcal*
- *Protein: 3.56 g*
- *Total Fat: 7.54 g*
- *Total Carbohydrates: 14.21 g*
- *Sodium: 599 mg*

58. Healthy Chicken Pasta Salad

Preparation time: 25 minutes

Cooking time: 20 minutes

Serving: 2

Difficulty level: Easy

Ingredients

- 8 oz whole wheat penne pasta
- 1 boneless, skinless chicken breast (6 oz)
- 1/2 cup low-fat plain Greek yogurt
- 1/4 cup walnut pieces
- 1/8 tsp (teaspoon) sea salt
- 1/2 tsp cracked black pepper
- 1 tbsp (tablespoon) red wine vinegar
- 1 cup seedless red grapes, halved
- 1/2 cup celery, chopped
- Olive oil, as needed

Directions:

1. Fill a large pot with water and bring to a boil. Add a splash of olive oil to prevent the pasta from sticking. Once boiling, add the penne pasta and cook for 8 to 10 minutes until al dente. Drain and set aside.
2. While the pasta is cooking, trim any excess fat from the chicken breast and cut it into small cubes. Place the chicken cubes in a medium-sized pot, ensuring they are covered with water. Bring to a boil over high heat and cook for 5 to 6 minutes.
3. Drain the cooked chicken.
4. In a large bowl, combine the cooked pasta, chicken, and the remaining ingredients. Mix well.
5. For the best flavor, refrigerate the salad for 20 to 30 minutes before serving.

Nutritional information

- *Calories: 115 kcal*
- *Total Fat: 4 g*
- *Protein: 10 g*
- *Total Carbohydrates: 11 g*
- *Sodium: 84 mg*

---

59. Broccoli Slaw

Preparation time: 10 minutes

Cooking time: 60 minutes

Serving: 2

Difficulty level: Easy

Ingredients

- 3 cups broccoli florets, blanched
- 1/4 cup carrot, shredded
- 2 tbsp (tablespoon) mayonnaise
- 1 tsp (teaspoon) Dijon mustard
- 1 tbsp red wine vinegar
- 1 tbsp shallots, minced
- 1/4 cup golden raisins
- 1/2 cup almonds, toasted and sliced
- Salt and pepper, to taste

Directions:

1. In a large bowl, combine all the ingredients.
2. Mix well until all ingredients are evenly coated.
3. Refrigerate the slaw for at least 60 minutes to allow the flavors to meld.
4. Serve chilled.

Nutritional information

- *Calories: 169.20 kcal*
- *Total Fat: 11.76 g*
- *Protein: 4.22 g*
- *Total Carbohydrates: 13.09 g*

60. Lentils with Rice and Onions

Preparation time: 15 minutes

Cooking time: 2 hour

Serving: 2

Difficulty level: Easy

Ingredients

- 1 1/2 cups green lentils, rinsed
- 3/4 cup brown basmati rice
- 3 large yellow onions, peeled and finely diced
- 3/4 tsp (teaspoon) ground cinnamon
- 1/2 tsp ground allspice
- 1 tbsp (tablespoon) salt
- Freshly ground black pepper, to taste
- 6 1/2 cups water

Directions:

1. In a large pot, combine lentils with 5 cups of water and bring to a boil over high heat. Reduce heat to medium and let simmer for 30 minutes.
2. Stir in the cinnamon and allspice, continuing to simmer for an additional 15 to 20 minutes.

3. In a separate medium saucepan, bring 1 1/2 cups of water to a boil. Add the rice, reduce heat to medium, cover, and cook for 45 minutes.
4. In a large skillet over high heat, sauté the onions, frequently stirring for 10 minutes. If the onions begin to stick, add water 1 tbsp at a time. Reduce heat to medium-low and continue cooking the onions for an additional 10 minutes.
5. Combine the lentils, rice, and onions in the skillet. Mix well and season with salt and freshly ground black pepper.

Nutritional information

- *Calories: 149 kcal*
- *Total Fat: 4.93 g*
- *Protein: 6.87 g*
- *Total Carbohydrates: 28.85 g*
- *Sodium: 9 mg*

61. Tabouli Salad

Preparation time: 4 hours 45 minutes

Cooking time: None

Serving: 2

Difficulty level: Medium

Ingredients

- 1/2 cup medium bulgur wheat
- 1 1/2 cups water
- 1/3 cup lemon juice
- 2 tbsp (tablespoon) fresh mint, chopped
- 1 tsp (teaspoon) salt
- 1 tsp black pepper
- 1/4 cup extra-virgin olive oil
- 1 cup fresh parsley, chopped
- 1/2 cup green onions, chopped
- 2 large tomatoes, diced
- 1 tbsp garlic, minced

Directions:

1. Soak the bulgur in water for a minimum of 2 hours.
2. After soaking, drain any excess water and transfer the bulgur to a large mixing bowl.
3. Add the lemon juice, mint, salt, pepper, olive oil, parsley, green onions, tomatoes, and minced garlic to the bowl. Mix thoroughly to combine.
4. Allow the salad to sit at room temperature for 60 minutes before serving. Alternatively, refrigerate overnight for enhanced flavor.
5. Serve either at room temperature or chilled, based on preference.

Preparing Your Bulgur:

1. Soak 2 cups of wheat berries in 4 cups of water overnight.
2. The next day, drain the soaked wheat berries and simmer them in 4 cups of water for 60 minutes.
3. After simmering, drain the wheat berries again and spread them out on a baking sheet.
4. Dry the wheat berries in an oven preheated to 250°F for about 45 minutes or until fully dried.
5. Once dried, process the wheat berries in a food processor until finely ground to achieve a bulgur-like consistency.
6. Store the prepared bulgur in an airtight container for future use.

Nutritional information

- *Calories: 141.52 kcal*
- *Total Fat: 9.69 g*
- *Protein: 2.34 g*
- *Total Carbohydrates: 12.95 g*

---

62. Carrot Salad

Preparation time: 10 minutes

Cooking time: None

Serving: 2

Difficulty level: Easy

Ingredients

- 1/2 cup salad oil
- 2 tbsp (tablespoon) honey mustard
- 1 tbsp white wine vinegar
- Salt, to taste
- Pepper, to taste
- 4 medium carrots
- 2 green onions

Directions:

1. In a blender, combine the salad oil, honey mustard, and vinegar. Blend until the mixture achieves a creamy consistency.
2. Season the dressing with salt and pepper according to your preference. Set the dressing aside.
3. Peel the carrots and shred them in a mixing bowl.
4. Thinly slice the green onions and add them to the shredded carrots.
5. Drizzle the prepared dressing over the carrot and onion mixture. Toss thoroughly to ensure even coating.
6. For optimal flavor, refrigerate the salad overnight before serving.

Nutritional information

- *Calories: 305.67 kcal*
- *Total Fat: 28.90 g*
- *Protein: 1.20 g*
- *Total Carbohydrates: 12.01 g*

63. Curried Shrimp Salad in a Papaya

Preparation time: 10 minutes

Cooking time: None

Serving: 2

Difficulty level: Easy

Ingredients

- 2 tbsp (tablespoon) olive oil
- 1 tbsp lemon juice
- 1 tsp (teaspoon) grated lemon zest
- 1/2 tsp curry powder
- Salt and pepper, to taste
- 1 cup cooked and peeled shrimp, chilled
- 1/4 cup diced celery
- 1/4 cup diced cucumber
- 1/4 cup seedless green grapes, halved
- 1 medium papaya
- 1/4 cup toasted sliced almonds

Directions:

1. In a mixing bowl, whisk together the olive oil, lemon juice, lemon zest, curry powder, salt, and pepper.
2. Add the shrimp, celery, cucumber, and grapes to the bowl. Toss the ingredients to ensure they are evenly coated with the dressing. Place the salad in the refrigerator to chill.
3. Halve the papaya lengthwise, ensuring you cut through the stem area. Carefully scoop out and discard the seeds.

4. Generously fill each papaya half with the chilled shrimp salad.

5. Garnish the top of the shrimp salad with toasted sliced almonds.

6. Serve the dish with both a fork and a spoon, allowing diners to scoop and enjoy the papaya flesh once the salad is consumed.

Nutritional information

- *Calories: 314.21 kcal*
- *Total Fat: 21.71 g*
- *Protein: 8.58 g*
- *Total Carbohydrates: 24.33 g*

64. Coconut and Almond Rice with Berries

Preparation time: 10 minutes

Cooking time: 30 minutes

Serving: 2

Difficulty level: Medium

Ingredients

- 1 cup brown basmati rice
- 2 dates, pitted and chopped
- 1 cup fresh blueberries (or raspberries), divided
- 1/4 cup toasted slivered almonds, divided
- 1/2 cup shaved coconut, divided
- 1 cup water
- 1 cup coconut milk
- 1 tsp (teaspoon) salt

Directions:

1. In a medium saucepan, combine the basmati rice, water, coconut milk, salt, and chopped dates. Place the saucepan over high heat.

2. Stir the mixture until it reaches a boil. Once boiling, reduce the heat to a simmer.

3. Allow the rice to cook for 20 to 30 minutes or until it becomes tender. Avoid stirring during this process.

4. Once cooked, divide the rice evenly among two bowls.

5. Garnish each bowl with half of the blueberries (or raspberries), almonds, and coconut.

6. Serve immediately.

Nutritional information

- *Calories: 281 kcal*
- *Total Fat: 8 g*
- *Protein: 6 g*
- *Total Carbohydrates: 49 g*
- *Sodium: 623 mg*

⚠ This recipe calls for coconut, which can be high in saturated fat. For individuals with heart conditions, it is advisable to limit the amount of coconut.

65. Zesty Rice with Cuban Black Beans

Preparation time: 20 minutes

Cooking time: 2 hours 30 minutes

Serving: 2

Difficulty level: Easy

Ingredients

For the Black Beans:

- 1 lb (pound) black beans, soaked overnight
- 1 large onion, diced
- 1 medium tomato, chopped
- 3 medium carrots, diced
- 1 red bell pepper, seeded and diced
- 5 cups water
- 2 bay leaves
- 3 garlic cloves, minced
- 3 celery stalks, diced
- 2 tbsp (tablespoons) ground cumin
- 2 tbsp minced oregano
- 1 cup cilantro stems, finely chopped
- 2 tbsp apple cider vinegar
- 1/2 tsp (teaspoon) freshly ground white or black pepper
- 3 tbsp cilantro leaves, chopped
- 1 tbsp salt

For the Cilantro Rice:

- 1 cup brown rice
- 2 tbsp cilantro leaves, finely chopped
- 1 tbsp low-sodium light brown miso paste
- 2 cups water

Directions:

For the Black Beans:

1. In a large pot, combine the beans, onion, cumin, garlic, bay leaves, celery, carrots, oregano, red pepper, cilantro stems, and 5 cups of water. Bring to a boil.
2. Reduce heat and simmer for 90 minutes.
3. Remove 1/4 of the beans, mash them in a separate bowl, and return them to the pot.

4. Stir in the apple cider vinegar, cilantro leaves, pepper, and tomato. Continue cooking until the beans are tender.
5. Season with salt and remove the bay leaves before serving.

For the Cilantro Rice:

1. In a large saucepan, bring the rice, miso paste, and 2 cups of water to a boil.
2. Reduce heat, cover, and simmer for 20 minutes.
3. Lower the heat further and continue to simmer for an additional 30 minutes.
4. Fluff the rice with a fork and stir in the chopped cilantro leaves.
5. To serve, divide the rice between two plates and top with the black beans.

Nutritional information

- *Calories: 642 kcal*
- *Total Fat: 4 g*
- *Protein: 31 g*
- *Total Carbohydrates: 123 g*
- *Sodium: 221 mg*

---

66. Vegan Fajita Bowl with Cabbage Rice

Preparation time: 10 minutes

Cooking time: 30 minutes

Serving: 2

Difficulty level: Medium

Ingredients

- Lime wedges for garnish
- 1/2 avocado, sliced
- 1/2 tsp (teaspoon) dried oregano
- 1/2 tsp garlic salt
- 1 small cauliflower, cut into florets
- 1 tbsp (tablespoon) chipotle paste
- 1 red bell pepper, sliced
- 1 tbsp fresh coriander (cilantro), chopped
- 1/2 tsp chili flakes
- 1/2 tsp smoked paprika
- 1/2 tsp cumin seeds
- 1 cup crushed tomatoes
- 1 red onion, sliced
- 1 tbsp olive oil
- Water, as needed

Directions:

1. In a frying pan, heat olive oil over medium heat. Add sliced peppers and onions, sautéing for 10 minutes.

2. Stir in the chipotle paste, a splash of water, and crushed tomatoes. Allow the mixture to simmer for 20 minutes.

3. In a food processor, pulse the cauliflower florets until they resemble grains.

4. In a separate pan, toast the cumin seeds briefly. Add the cauliflower "rice" to the pan along with smoked paprika, chili flakes, garlic salt, and oregano. Sauté for 6 minutes. Season with black pepper and additional salt, if desired.

5. To serve, divide the cauliflower rice between two bowls. Top with the pepper and onion mixture, avocado slices, and chopped cilantro. Garnish with lime wedges.

Nutritional information

- *Calories: 174 kcal*
- *Total Fat: 4.4 g*
- *Protein: 7 g*
- *Total Carbohydrates: 22.1 g*
- *Sodium: 9 mg*

4.7 Vegetarian and Vegan Culinary Creations

67. Vegetarian Bolognese

Preparation time: 10 minutes

Cooking time: 45 minutes

Serving: 2

Difficulty level: Medium

Ingredients

- Grana Padano or a vegetarian alternative, grated, to taste
- 33.8 oz (1 liter) vegetable broth
- 1 tsp (teaspoon) dried oregano
- 2 cups crushed tomatoes
- 1 cup button mushrooms, sliced
- 2 garlic cloves, minced
- 2 carrots, diced
- 2 tbsp (tablespoon) olive oil
- 1 1/2 cups tagliatelle pasta
- 2 bay leaves
- 3 tbsp tomato puree
- 1 1/2 cups puy lentils, rinsed
- 1/2 tsp dried chili flakes
- 2 celery stalks, diced
- 1 large onion, diced

Directions:

1. In a large frying pan, heat olive oil over medium heat. Add celery, onion, dried chili flakes, garlic, carrots, and mushrooms. Sauté until the vegetables are softened.

2. Stir in the lentils, tomato puree, vegetable broth, bay leaves, oregano, and crushed tomatoes. Bring the mixture to a boil, then reduce the heat and let it simmer for 45 minutes or until the lentils are tender.

3. While the sauce is simmering, cook the tagliatelle pasta according to the package instructions. Drain and set aside.

4. Serve the bolognese sauce over the cooked tagliatelle. Garnish with grated Grana Padano or its vegetarian alternative.

Nutritional information

- *Calories: 394 kcal*
- *Total Fat: 8.1 g*
- *Protein: 23.7 g*
- *Total Carbohydrates: 49.2 g*
- *Sodium: 27 mg*

68. Vegetable Kabobs

Preparation time: 25 minutes

Cooking time: 12 minutes

Serving: 2

Difficulty level: Hard

Ingredients

- 2 tbsp (tablespoon) olive oil
- 2 garlic cloves, minced
- Juice of 1/2 lemon
- 1/2 tsp (teaspoon) dried oregano
- 1/2 tsp dried basil
- Salt, to taste
- Freshly ground black pepper, to taste
- 1 cup cremini mushrooms, cleaned
- 1/2 cup cherry tomatoes
- 1 green bell pepper, cut into chunks
- 1 red onion, cut into chunks
- 1 yellow squash, cut into thick rounds

Directions:

1. Preheat the oven to 400°F (204°C).
2. In a mixing bowl, combine olive oil, minced garlic, lemon juice, oregano, and basil. Season with salt and freshly ground black pepper, and mix well.
3. Thread the mushrooms, tomatoes, bell pepper, onion, and squash onto skewers. Arrange the skewers on a baking sheet.
4. Generously brush the vegetables with the prepared oil mixture. Allow them to marinate for 10 to 15 minutes.
5. Roast in the preheated oven for 10 to 12 minutes or until the vegetables are tender.
6. Serve the kabobs immediately.

Nutritional information

- *Calories: 191 kcal*
- *Total Fat: 15 g*
- *Total Carbohydrates: 15 g*
- *Protein: 4 g*

69. Perfect Sweet Potatoes

Preparation time: 5 minutes

Cooking time: 7 to 8 hours

Serving: 2

Difficulty level: Easy

Ingredients

- 6 sweet potatoes, thoroughly washed and dried

Directions:

1. Crumple 7 to 8 pieces of aluminum foil into loose balls and arrange them at the bottom of a 6-quart slow cooker, covering approximately half of its surface.
2. Using a fork, pierce each sweet potato 6 to 8 times. Wrap each potato individually in aluminum foil, ensuring it's fully sealed.
3. Place the wrapped sweet potatoes atop the foil balls in the slow cooker.
4. Cover the slow cooker and set it to low. Allow the sweet potatoes to cook for 7 to 8 hours.
5. Using tongs, carefully remove the sweet potatoes from the slow cooker. Let them cool for a few minutes before unwrapping the foil. Serve while still warm.

Nutritional information

- *Calories: 129 kcal*
- *Total Fat: 0 g*
- *Total Carbohydrates: 30 g*
- *Protein: 2 g*

70. Roasted Red Pepper Hummus

Preparation time: 5 minutes

Cooking time: None

Serving: 2

Difficulty level: Medium

Ingredients

- 2 cups chickpeas
- 1 cup red bell pepper, roughly chopped
- 2 tbsp sesame seeds
- 1 tbsp fresh lemon juice
- 1 tbsp olive oil
- 1/4 tsp ground cumin
- 1 tsp onion powder
- 1 tsp garlic powder
- 1 tsp salt
- 1/4 tsp freshly ground black pepper

Directions:

1. Combine all ingredients in a blender or food processor.
2. Blend until a smooth and creamy consistency is achieved.
3. Transfer the hummus to a serving bowl.

Nutritional information

- Calories: 45 kcal
- Total Fat: 2 g (grams)
- Total Carbohydrates: 6 g (grams)
- Protein: 2 g (grams)
- Sodium: 190 mg (milligrams)

71. Roasted Potatoes with Herbs

Preparation time: 10 minutes

Cooking time: 25 minutes

Serving: 2

Difficulty level: Easy

Ingredients

- 3/4 lb (pounds) potatoes, cubed
- 4 garlic cloves, finely chopped
- 2 tsp olive oil
- 2 tsp fresh rosemary, finely chopped
- 1/8 tsp salt
- 1/4 tsp freshly ground black pepper
- 2 tsp unsalted butter
- 2 tbsp fresh parsley, finely chopped
- Cooking spray

Directions:

1. Preheat the oven to 400°F (degrees Fahrenheit).
2. Lightly coat a baking dish with cooking spray.
3. In a mixing bowl, combine the cubed potatoes, garlic, olive oil, rosemary, salt, and black pepper. Toss to ensure

the potatoes are well-coated with the mixture.

4. Transfer the coated potatoes to the prepared baking dish and cover them with aluminum foil.

5. Bake in the preheated oven for 25 minutes or until the potatoes are golden brown and tender.

6. Before serving, top the roasted potatoes with butter and sprinkle with chopped parsley.

Nutritional information

- *Calories: 104 kcal*
- *Total Fat: 4 g*
- *Total Carbohydrates: 15 g*
- *Protein: 2 g*
- *Sodium: 103 mg*

72. Spiced Eggplant Fritters

Preparation time: 15 minutes

Cooking time: 20 minutes

Serving: 2

Difficulty level: Medium

Ingredients

- 2 eggplants, sliced into 0.4-inch-thick rounds
- 1/2 cup all-purpose flour, seasoned
- 1 tsp ground sumac
- 2 large eggs
- 2 cups panko breadcrumbs
- 2 spring onions (green onions), thinly sliced
- 1 cup red vein sorrel (for garnish)
- Olive oil (for shallow frying)
- 1 cup thick Greek-style yogurt
- Juice of 1 lemon
- 1 garlic clove, minced
- 4 heirloom tomatoes, sliced
- Seeds from 1 pomegranate
- 2 tsp sea salt flakes

Directions:

1. Sprinkle the eggplant slices with 2 tsp of sea salt flakes and place them in a colander set over a bowl. Allow them to sit for 30 minutes to draw out any bitterness.

2. Rinse the eggplant slices under cold water and pat dry with paper towels.

3. In a mixing bowl, combine the flour and sumac.

4. In a separate bowl, lightly beat the eggs.

5. Place the panko breadcrumbs in a third bowl.

6. Dip each eggplant slice first into the flour mixture, then into the beaten eggs (allowing any excess to drip off), and finally coat with the panko breadcrumbs.

7. Heat the olive oil in a large, non-stick frying pan over medium heat. Fry the

eggplant slices in batches for 5 to 6 minutes on each side or until they are golden brown and tender. Keep them warm as you continue with the remaining slices.

8. In a separate bowl, mix the Greek yogurt, lemon juice, and minced garlic. Season to taste.

9. To serve, arrange the fried eggplant slices on a platter and top with sliced tomatoes, pomegranate seeds, sliced spring onions, and red vein sorrel. Serve immediately with the yogurt mixture on the side.

Nutritional information

- *Calories: 201 kcal*
- *Total Fat: 5.1 g*
- *Protein: 13.1 g*
- *Total Carbohydrates: 21.9 g*
- *Sodium: 14 mg*

73. Broccoli Rice Casserole

Preparation time: 10 minutes

Cooking time: 60 minutes

Serving: 2

Difficulty level: Easy

Ingredients

- 1 1/2 cups wild rice
- 6 cups broccoli florets
- 2 cups reduced-sodium cream of mushroom soup
- 2 cups low-fat cheddar cheese, shredded

Directions:

1. Preheat the oven to 325°F (163°C).

2. Cook the wild rice according to the package instructions.

3. Once cooked, spread the rice evenly at the bottom of a 9 x 9-inch (23 x 23 cm) casserole dish.

4. Steam the broccoli florets for 5 minutes until they are slightly tender but still vibrant in color.

5. Layer the steamed broccoli over the rice in the casserole dish.

6. In a separate bowl, mix the reduced-sodium cream of mushroom soup and shredded cheddar cheese. Spread this mixture over the broccoli layer.

7. Place the casserole dish in the preheated oven and bake uncovered for 45 minutes or until the top is golden and bubbly.

Nutritional information

- *Calories: 293 kcal*
- *Total Fat: 5 g*
- *Protein: 20 g*
- *Total Carbohydrates: 44 g*

⚠ Readers with cardiovascular conditions should be aware that this dish contains low-fat cheddar cheese, which may contribute to the intake of saturated fats and sodium. In the interest of cardiac health, it is advisable to substitute low-fat cheddar cheese with a heart-healthier option. Low-fat ricotta or cottage cheese are recommended alternatives due to their lower saturated fat and sodium content. For individuals adhering to a plant-based diet or those with lactose intolerance, nut or seed-based vegan cheese alternatives can be used to provide beneficial unsaturated fats, contributing to a more heart-healthy profile.

74. Cabbage Pilaf

Preparation time: 10 minutes

Cooking time: 50 minutes

Serving: 2

Difficulty level: Medium

Ingredients

- 2 1/4 cups low-sodium vegetable broth
- 3/4 cup millet
- 1 medium carrot, peeled and diced
- 1 medium leek (white and light green parts only), diced and thoroughly rinsed
- 1 celery stalk, diced
- 2 garlic cloves, minced
- 3 cups cabbage, chopped
- 1 tsp fresh thyme, minced
- 1 tbsp fresh dill, minced
- Salt and freshly ground black pepper to taste

Directions:

1. In a medium saucepan, bring the vegetable broth to a boil over high heat. Stir in the millet and return to a boil. Reduce the heat to medium-low, cover, and simmer for 20 minutes or until the millet is tender and the broth is absorbed.
2. In a separate large saucepan, sauté the carrot, leek, and celery over medium heat for 7 to 8 minutes. If the vegetables start to stick, add water, a tablespoon at a time.
3. Stir in the garlic, dill, thyme, and cabbage. Continue to cook over medium heat for approximately 10 minutes, stirring frequently, until the cabbage is tender.
4. Add the cooked millet to the vegetable mixture and stir well. Continue cooking for an additional 5 minutes, stirring often. Season with salt and freshly ground black pepper to taste.

Nutritional information

- *Calories: 219 kcal*
- *Total Carbohydrates: 44.27 g*
- *Protein: 7.32 g*
- *Sodium: 118 mg*

75. Cauliflower-cream pasta with Mint

Preparation time: 15 minutes

Cooking time: 30 minutes

Serving: 2

Difficulty level: Easy

Ingredients

- 1 medium cauliflower head, separated into florets
- 2 cups low-sodium vegetable broth
- 1 zucchini, peeled and diced
- 1 small acorn squash, peeled, halved, seeded, and cut into 1/2-inch cubes
- 1 lb whole-grain penne pasta, cooked as per package instructions and drained
- 1 medium red bell pepper, seeded and diced
- 3 garlic cloves, minced
- 3 sprigs of mint, finely chopped
- Salt and freshly ground black pepper to taste

Directions:

1. In a medium saucepan, combine the cauliflower and vegetable broth. Bring to a boil over medium heat and cook for about 10 minutes or until the cauliflower is tender.
2. Remove from heat and transfer the mixture to a food processor. Blend until it achieves a smooth, creamy consistency. Set aside.
3. In a large saucepan, sauté the zucchini and red bell pepper over medium heat for 7 to 8 minutes. If the vegetables start to stick, add water, a tablespoon at a time.
4. Stir in the garlic, mint, and acorn squash. Continue cooking for an additional 5 to 6 minutes or until the squash is tender.
5. Add the cauliflower purée and the cooked penne pasta to the saucepan. Toss to combine thoroughly. Season with salt and freshly ground black pepper to taste.

Nutritional information

- *Calories: 232 kcal*
- *Total Carbohydrates: 47.43 g*
- *Protein: 10.64 g*
- *Fat: 2.1 g*
- *Sodium: 543 mg*

76. Potato and Vegetable Casserole

Preparation time: 10 minutes

Cooking time: 30 minutes

Serving: 2

Difficulty level: Medium

Ingredients

- 6 potatoes
- 2 tbsp olive oil
- 1 cup onion, thinly sliced
- 2 cups cabbage, coarsely chopped
- 2 cups cauliflower florets, coarsely chopped
- 1 tsp garlic, minced
- 1 cup fat-free plain yogurt
- 2 cups canned white kidney beans, drained and rinsed
- 1/4 cup fresh dill, finely chopped
- 1/2 tsp paprika

Directions:

1. Preheat the oven to 325°F.

2. Boil the potatoes until they are almost fully cooked. Allow them to cool slightly, then peel if desired.

3. In a large skillet, heat the olive oil over medium-high heat. Add the onions and sauté until translucent.

4. Incorporate the cabbage, cauliflower, and garlic into the skillet. Continue to sauté until the vegetables are tender.

5. Stir in the yogurt, followed by the rinsed white kidney beans. Mix well and remove from heat.

6. Slice the cooled potatoes into rounds. Layer half of the potato slices at the bottom of a 9 x 13-inch (23 x 33 cm) baking dish that has been lightly coated with nonstick spray.

7. Evenly spread the vegetable and bean mixture over the layer of potatoes.

8. Top with the remaining potato slices.

9. Garnish the casserole with chopped dill and a sprinkle of paprika.

10. Bake in the preheated oven for 20 minutes.

Nutritional information

- *Calories: 462 kcal*
- *Total Carbohydrates: 88 g*
- *Protein: 17 g*
- *Fat: 6 g*

⚠ This recipe includes potatoes, which are high in carbohydrates. Individuals with cardiac concerns, particularly those also managing blood glucose levels, should consume such dishes in moderation. Additionally, while olive oil and fat-free yogurt are heart-healthier options, portion control is recommended to maintain a balanced diet.

77. Root Vegetable Curry

Preparation time: 10 minutes

Cooking time: 20 minutes

Serving: 2

Difficulty level: Easy

Ingredients

- 1 tsp olive oil
- 2 shallots, finely diced
- 1/2 tsp garlic, minced
- 1 tbsp curry powder or paste
- 1 parsnip, peeled and cut into 1-inch chunks
- 1 sweet potato, peeled and diced into 1-inch pieces
- 1 carrot, peeled and cut into 1-inch chunks
- 1 cup canned lentils, drained and rinsed
- 1 tomato, finely chopped
- 1/2 cup low-sodium vegetable stock

Directions:

1. In a large saucepan, heat the olive oil over medium-high heat. Add the shallots and garlic, sautéing until they become translucent, approximately 2 minutes.

2. Stir in the curry powder or paste, continuing to sauté for an additional minute.

3. Incorporate the parsnip, sweet potato, carrot, lentils, tomato, and vegetable stock into the saucepan.

4. Bring the mixture to a boil, then reduce the heat to low. Allow the curry to simmer until the root vegetables are tender, which should take around 15 minutes.

Nutritional information

- *Calories: 321 kcal*
- *Total Carbohydrates: 57.9 g*
- *Protein: 16.5 g*
- *Fat: 4.3 g*
- *Sodium: 88 mg*

78. Veggie Burger with Spice Medley

Preparation time: 10 minutes

Cooking time: 20 minutes

Serving: 2

Difficulty level: Medium

Ingredients

- 1 tbsp black pepper (adjust to taste)
- 3 tbsp plain flour
- 2 tsp thyme
- 2 tsp parsley
- 2 tsp garlic, minced
- 2 tsp melted coconut oil
- 2 tsp chives
- 1 tsp mustard powder
- 1 flax egg (1 tbsp ground flaxseed combined with 3 tbsp water)
- 1 cup breadcrumbs
- 1/2 lb cauliflower, steamed and finely diced
- 1/2 cup oats
- 1/4 cup desiccated coconut

Directions:

1. Preheat the oven to 400°F (204°C).
2. Set an oven-safe wire rack atop a baking sheet. Lightly coat the wire rack with non-stick cooking spray.
3. Using a tea towel, wring out any excess water from the steamed cauliflower. Transfer the cauliflower to a mixing bowl.
4. To the bowl, add all the ingredients, excluding the breadcrumbs. Mix thoroughly until well combined.
5. Shape the mixture into 8 burger patties using your hands.
6. Coat each patty in breadcrumbs and position them on the prepared wire rack.
7. Bake in the oven for 10 minutes. Flip the patties and continue baking for an additional 5 to 10 minutes or until they achieve a light brown, crisp finish.
8. Serve immediately.

Nutritional information

- *Calories: 121 kcal*
- *Total Carbohydrates: 17.4 g*
- *Protein: 4.3 g*
- *Fat: 3.8 g*
- *Sodium: 49 mg*

⚠ Note that this recipe calls for coconut oil, a source of saturated fat. For those with heart disease, the American Heart Association recommends minimizing the intake of saturated fats to reduce the risk of heart disease. Consider substituting with an oil high in unsaturated fats, such as olive oil.

4.8   Desserts: Indulgence   without   Guilt

79. Banana Strawberry Muffins

Preparation time: 10 minutes

Cooking time: 35 minutes

Serving: 2

Difficulty level: Hard

Ingredients

- 2 eggs
- 3 ripe bananas, mashed
- 1/2 cup unsweetened applesauce
- 2 cups whole wheat flour
- 1/4 cup vegetable oil
- 1 tsp baking soda
- 3/4 cup packed brown sugar
- 1 tbsp ground cinnamon
- 1 tsp vanilla extract
- 1 cup frozen sliced strawberries

Directions:

1. Preheat the oven to 375°F (190°C). Prepare 12 muffin cups by greasing them or lining them with paper liners.
2. In a large mixing bowl, whisk together the eggs, applesauce, oil, brown sugar, vanilla extract, and mashed bananas.
3. In a separate bowl, combine the whole wheat flour, baking soda, and ground cinnamon.
4. Gradually incorporate the dry ingredients into the banana mixture until just moistened.
5. Gently fold in the frozen sliced strawberries, ensuring they are evenly distributed throughout the batter.
6. Evenly distribute the batter among the prepared muffin cups.
7. Bake in the preheated oven for approximately 20 minutes or until the tops of the muffins spring back when lightly pressed.
8. Allow the muffins to cool in the tin for a few minutes before transferring them to a wire rack to cool completely.

Nutritional information

- *Calories: 212 kcal*
- *Total Carbohydrates: 38.1 g*
- *Fat: 5.9 g*
- *Protein: 4.2 g*

⚠ Attention is warranted for the inclusion of vegetable oil and brown sugar in this recipe. Those with cardiovascular health concerns should be cautious about the intake of added sugars and fats. Opting for substitutions such as unsweetened applesauce for oil and reducing the sugar content may be beneficial.

---

80. Ricotta Stuffed Peaches

Preparation time: 10 minutes

Cooking time: 5 minutes

Serving: 2

Difficulty level: Easy

Ingredients

- 4 peaches, pitted and halved
- 2 tbsp ricotta cheese
- 2 tbsp liquid honey
- 3/4 cup water
- 1/2 tsp vanilla extract
- 3/4 tsp ground cinnamon
- 1 tbsp sliced almonds
- 3/4 tsp saffron threads

Directions:

1. In a saucepan, bring 3/4 cup of water to a boil.
2. Stir in the vanilla extract, saffron, ground cinnamon, and liquid honey until the honey dissolves and the mixture is fragrant. Then remove from heat.
3. Gently place the peach halves into the aromatic honey liquid, ensuring they are coated.
4. In a separate bowl, combine the ricotta cheese, a dash of vanilla extract, and sliced almonds to create the filling.
5. Once the peaches have been infused with the honey mixture, arrange them on a serving plate.
6. Spoon the ricotta mixture into the cavity of each peach half.
7. Top each filled peach half with its corresponding half to form a whole peach again.
8. Drizzle the peaches with the remaining honey mixture before serving.

Nutritional information

- *Calories: 177 kcal*
- *Total Fat: 9.5 g*
- *Sodium: 20 mg*
- *Total Carbohydrates: 21.4 g*
- *Protein: 5.9 g*

81. Sweet Potato and Pumpkin Pie

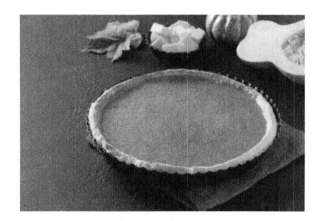

Preparation time: 10 minutes

Cooking time: 60 minutes

Serving: 2

Difficulty level: Easy

Ingredients

- 1 sweet potato, peeled and cooked (weight after cooking: approximately 8 oz)
- 1 buttercup squash, peeled, seeded, and cooked (weight after cooking: approximately 8 oz)
- 1/2 cup silken tofu
- 1/2 cup soy milk
- 1/4 cup egg whites
- 1/4 cup rye flour (approximately 1 oz)
- 1/2 tsp ground cloves
- 1/2 tsp ground cinnamon
- 1/2 tsp ground nutmeg
- 1/2 tsp vanilla extract
- 1 tsp freshly grated ginger
- 1 tsp orange zest
- 3 tbsp honey
- 1 frozen pre-made 9-inch pie shell

Directions:

1. Preheat the oven to 300°F (150°C).
2. In a food processor, purée the cooked sweet potato and buttercup squash until smooth.
3. Transfer the purée to a large mixing bowl.
4. Incorporate the silken tofu, soy milk, egg whites, rye flour, spices, vanilla extract, grated ginger, orange zest, and honey into the purée, mixing until achieving a uniform consistency.
5. Place the pre-made pie shell on a baking sheet to catch any potential spills.
6. Pour the mixture into the pie shell, ensuring an even distribution.
7. Bake in the preheated oven for 45 to 55 minutes or until the pie reaches an internal temperature of 180°F (82°C), indicating that it is fully set.

Nutritional information

- *Calories: 210 kcal*
- *Protein: 5 g*
- *Total Carbohydrates: 34 g*
- *Total Fat: 6 g*
- *Sodium: 109 mg*

⚠ Although sweet potatoes and pumpkin are nutrient-dense choices, the addition of honey contributes additional sugars. Furthermore, the use of a pre-made pie shell may introduce trans fats, depending on the product. Readers are advised to check for trans fat content and consider homemade alternatives using whole grain flours and minimal added sugars

82. Apple-Berry Cobbler

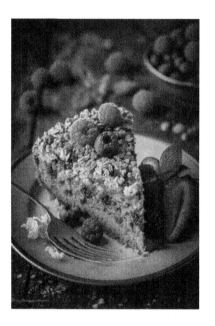

Preparation time: 55 minutes

Cooking time: 40 minutes

Serving: 2

Difficulty level: Easy

Ingredients

- 1 cup fresh raspberries (approximately 4 oz)
- 1 cup fresh blueberries (approximately 4 oz)
- 2 cups chopped apples (approximately 8 oz)
- 2 tbsp Turbinado or brown sugar
- 1/2 tsp ground cinnamon
- 1 tsp lemon zest
- 2 tsp lemon juice
- 1 1/2 tbsp cornstarch

Ingredients for the Topping:

- 1 large egg white
- 1/4 cup soy milk
- 1/4 tsp salt
- 1/2 tsp vanilla extract
- 1 1/2 tbsp Turbinado or brown sugar
- 3/4 cup whole-wheat pastry flour (approximately 3 oz)

Directions:

1. Preheat the oven to 350°F (175°C).
2. Apply a light coating of cooking spray to six individual oven-safe ramekins.
3. In a medium bowl, combine raspberries, blueberries, chopped apples, sugar, lemon juice, lemon zest, and cinnamon. Stir to distribute ingredients evenly.
4. Sprinkle cornstarch over the fruit mixture and stir to incorporate thoroughly. Set aside.
5. In a separate bowl, whisk the egg white until frothy.
6. To the egg white, add soy milk, vanilla extract, sugar, salt, and whole-wheat pastry flour. Stir until the mixture is well combined.
7. Evenly distribute the fruit mixture among the prepared ramekins.
8. Spoon the topping mixture over the fruit in each ramekin.
9. Place ramekins on a baking sheet to catch any drips and bake in the preheated oven for approximately 30 minutes or until the topping is golden brown and the filling is bubbling.

Nutritional information

- *Calories: 119 kcal*
- *Protein: 3.5 g*
- *Total Carbohydrates: 24 g*
- *Total Fat: 0 g*
- *Sodium: 114 mg*

---

83. Fruit Compote

Preparation time: 10 minutes

Cooking time: 20 minutes

Serving: 2

Difficulty level: Medium

Ingredients

- 1/4 cups water
- 1 cup orange juice (approximately 8 oz)
- 15 oz dried mixed fruit
- 2 tsp ground cinnamon
- 1/4 tsp ground nutmeg
- 1/4 tsp fresh ginger, crushed

Directions:

1. Combine water, orange juice, dried fruit, cinnamon, nutmeg, and ginger in a saucepan.
2. Stir the mixture and bring to a simmer over low heat.
3. Cover the saucepan with a lid and allow the compote to simmer for 10 minutes.
4. Remove the lid and continue to simmer for an additional 10 minutes, allowing the flavors to concentrate and the liquid to reduce slightly.

Nutritional information

- *Calories: 208 kcal*
- *Total Fat: 0 g*
- *Total Carbohydrates: 47 g*
- *Protein: 5 g*
- *Sodium: 68 mg*

84. Creamy Delicious Farro

Preparation time: 10 minutes

Cooking time: 30 minutes

Serving: 2

Difficulty level: Easy

Ingredients

- 1 cup farro (approximately 7.1 oz or 200 grams), rinsed and drained
- 6 dates (approximately 1.4 oz or 40 grams), pitted and chopped
- 1/2 tsp ground cardamom
- 1 tsp vanilla extract
- 2 cups water
- 1 cup unsweetened soy milk or almond milk (approximately 8 fl oz)

Directions:

1. In a medium saucepan, bring water and soy milk to a boil over high heat.
2. Stir in the farro, chopped dates, cardamom powder, and vanilla extract.
3. Reduce heat to low and simmer for 25 to 30 minutes, or until the farro is tender and the mixture has thickened to a creamy consistency, stirring occasionally.
4. Serve the farro warm, allowing the flavors to meld together.

Nutritional information

- *Calories: 142 kcal*
- *Total Fat: 5 g*
- *Total Carbohydrates: 22.1 g*
- *Protein: 4.6 g*

⚠ While farro is a whole grain and beneficial for heart health, the addition of dairy can introduce saturated fats. Consider using unsweetened almond milk or soy milk as a substitute for dairy to reduce saturated fat intake.

85. Brown Rice Pudding

Preparation time: 10 minutes

Cooking time: 4 hour

Serving: 2

Difficulty level: Easy

Ingredients

- 1/2 cup brown rice (approximately 3.5 oz or 100 grams), rinsed
- 1/4 cup raisins (approximately 1.3 oz or 36 grams)
- 1/4 cup walnuts (approximately 1 oz or 30 grams), chopped
- 1 1/2 tsp ground cinnamon
- 2 tbsp agave syrup (approximately 1.4 oz or 40 ml)
- 1 tsp vanilla extract
- 1 1/2 cups unsweetened almond milk (approximately 12 fl oz or 355 ml)
- 1 1/2 cups unsweetened coconut milk or almond milk (approximately 12 fl oz or 355 ml)
- A pinch of salt

Directions:

1. Combine the brown rice, chopped walnuts, ground cinnamon, agave syrup, vanilla extract, almond milk, coconut milk, and a pinch of salt in a slow cooker. Stir the mixture thoroughly to ensure an even distribution of ingredients.
2. Cover the slow cooker and set it to cook on low heat for 4 hours.
3. After 4 hours, add the raisins to the mixture, stirring well to incorporate.
4. Serve the pudding warm, garnished as desired.

Nutritional information

- *Calories: 401 kcal*
- *Total Fat: 26.5 g*
- *Total Carbohydrates: 39.8 g*
- *Protein: 5.8 g*

⚠ This dessert contains coconut milk, which is high in saturated fats. It is recommended to make this dish more suitable for those with heart conditions to replace coconut milk with unsweetened almond milk or oat milk. These substitutes offer a lower saturated fat content and are considered more heart-healthy while still maintaining the desired creamy texture of the pudding.

---

86. Watermelon Wedges with Lemon

Preparation time: 10 minutes

Cooking time: None

Serving: 2

Difficulty level: Easy

Ingredients

- 1/2 cup freshly squeezed lemon juice (approximately 4 oz or 120 ml)
- 3 tbsp honey (approximately 1.5 oz or 45 ml)
- 3-inch-thick slices of chilled watermelon quartered (weight will vary)

Directions:

1. Whisk together the freshly squeezed lemon juice and honey in a mixing bowl until well combined.
2. Arrange the watermelon wedges on a serving platter and drizzle the lemon and honey mixture over the top.
3. Serve the watermelon wedges immediately while chilled for a refreshing treat.

Nutritional information

- *Calories: 222 kcal*
- *Total Protein: 0.3 g*
- *Total Carbohydrates: 61 g*
- *Total Fat: 0.7 g*
- *Sodium: 4 mg*

87. Cherry Stew

Preparation time: 25 minutes

Cooking time: 10 minutes

Serving: 2

Difficulty level: Easy

Ingredients

- 1/2 cup cocoa powder (approximately 1.6 oz or 45 g)
- 1 lb cherries, pitted (16 oz or 454 g)
- 1 cup coconut sugar (approximately 7.1 oz or 200 g)
- 2 cups water (16 fl oz or 473 ml)

Directions:

1. Combine the pitted cherries, water, coconut sugar, and cocoa powder in a saucepan.
2. Stir the mixture and cook over medium heat for 10 minutes, ensuring the sugar dissolves and the cherries soften.
3. Once cooked, allow the stew to cool to room temperature. Then, refrigerate until cold.
4. Divide the chilled cherry stew into bowls and serve as a refreshing dessert.

Nutritional information

- *Calories: 207 kcal*
- *Total Fat: 1 g (grams)*
- *Dietary Fiber: 3 g (grams)*
- *Protein: 6 g (grams)*

4.9 Beverages: Nutritious Smoothies and Juices

88. Strawberry Cocoa Smoothie

Preparation time: 5 minutes

Cooking time: 0 minutes

Serving: 2

Difficulty level: Medium

Ingredients

- 1 tbsp honey (21g)
- 1 1/2 cups frozen strawberries (approximately 210g)
- 1 tbsp unsweetened cocoa powder (5g)
- 1 cup chilled unsweetened almond milk (240ml)

Directions:

1. Combine honey, frozen strawberries, cocoa powder, and chilled almond milk in a blender.
2. Process the mixture until it achieves a smooth consistency.
3. Serve immediately for optimal freshness and flavor.

Nutritional information

- *Calories: 152*
- *Fat: 1.5 g*
- *Sodium: 91 mg*
- *Carbohydrates: 35.5 g*
- *Protein: 2.5 g*

⚠ The original recipe included unsalted butter, which has been omitted in this edited version to better align with dietary recommendations for individuals with cardiac concerns. Butter, even unsalted, is high in saturated fats, which can contribute to heart disease. The revised recipe maintains flavor while promoting heart health.

89. Peanut Strawberry Smoothie

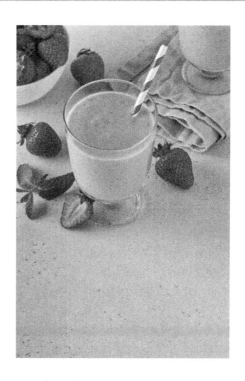

Preparation time: 10 minutes

Cooking time: 0 minutes

Serving: 2

Difficulty level: Easy

Ingredients

- 2–4 ice cubes (optional for texture)
- 1 tbsp honey (0.75 oz or 21g)
- 1 cup chopped kale, stems removed (2.4 oz or 67g)
- 1 cup unsweetened soy milk (8 fl oz or 240ml)
- 1 tsp vanilla extract (0.14 oz or 4.2g)
- 1 tbsp natural peanut butter, no added salt or sugar (0.56 oz or 16g)
- 1 cup frozen strawberries (5.36 oz or 152g)

Directions:

1. Place ice cubes (if using), honey, kale, soy milk, vanilla extract, peanut butter, and frozen strawberries into a blender.
2. Blend the mixture until it reaches a creamy consistency.
3. Serve immediately to enjoy the full flavor and nutritional benefits.

Nutritional information

- *Calories: 235*
- *Fat: 8.5 g*
- *Sodium: 95 mg*
- *Carbohydrates: 34 g*
- *Protein: 10 g*

90. Apple Tart Smoothie

Preparation time: 5 minutes

Cooking time: 0 minutes

Serving: 2

Difficulty level: Easy

Ingredients

- 1 red apple, chopped and frozen (approx. 182g / 6.4 oz US / 0.4 lb US)
- 2 cups chopped Boston lettuce (approx. 178g / 6.3 oz US / 0.39 lb US)
- 1 avocado, chopped and frozen (approx. 201g / 7.1 oz US / 0.44 lb US)
- 1/2 cup walnuts (approx. 59g / 2.1 oz US / 0.13 lb US)
- 1 tbsp apple cider vinegar (approx. 14.9ml / 0.5 fl oz US / 15g)
- 1 1/2 cups water (approx. 355ml / 12 fl oz US)

Directions:

1. In a high-powered blender, combine the frozen apple, Boston lettuce, frozen avocado, walnuts, apple cider vinegar, and water.
2. Blend on high speed until the mixture is smooth.
3. Pour the smoothie evenly into two cups and serve immediately.

Nutritional information

- *Calories: 407*
- *Fat: 34.1g*
- *Carbohydrates: 26.4g*
- *Protein: 7.4g*
- *Sodium: 11.3mg*

91. Kiwi, Zucchini, and Pear Smoothie

Preparation time: 5 minutes

Cooking time: 0 minutes

Serving: 2

Difficulty level: Medium

Ingredients

- 2 kiwis, peeled, chopped, and frozen (approx. 148g / 5.2 oz US / 0.33 lb US)
- 1 cup chopped zucchini (approx. 124g / 4.4 oz US / 0.27 lb US)
- 1 pear, chopped and frozen (approx. 178g / 6.3 oz US / 0.39 lb US)
- 1 cup fresh spinach (approx. 30g / 1 oz US / 0.06 lb US)
- 1 1/2 cups unsweetened almond milk (approx. 355ml / 12 fl oz US)

Directions:

1. Combine the frozen kiwis, chopped zucchini, frozen pear, fresh spinach, and unsweetened almond milk in a blender.
2. Blend on high until the mixture achieves a smooth consistency.
3. Pour the smoothie into two cups, distributing evenly, and serve immediately.

Nutritional information

- *Calories: 121*
- *Fat: 3g*
- *Carbohydrates: 23.4g*
- *Protein: 3.3g*
- *Sodium: 165mg*

92. Green Mango Smoothie

Preparation time: 5 minutes

Cooking time: 0 minutes

Serving: 2

Difficulty level: Easy

Ingredients

- 1 cup frozen mango chunks (approx. 165g / 5.8 oz US / 0.36 lb US)
- 2 cups chopped radish greens (approx. 128g / 4.5 oz US / 0.28 lb US)
- 1 avocado, peeled and pitted (approx. 200g / 7 oz US / 0.44 lb US)
- 2 tbsp chia seeds (approx. 24g / 0.85 oz US / 0.05 lb US)
- 1 cup full-fat plain Greek yogurt (approx. 245g / 8.6 oz US / 0.54 lb US)
- 1 1/2 cups water (approx. 355ml / 12 fl oz US)

Directions:

1. In a blender, combine the frozen mango chunks, chopped radish greens, peeled and pitted avocado, chia seeds, full-fat plain Greek yogurt, and water. Blend on high until the mixture is smooth.
2. Serve the smoothie equally in two cups.

Nutritional information

- *Calories: 440*
- *Fat: 26.8g*

- *Carbohydrates: 37g*
- *Protein: 17.4g*
- *Sodium: 88.3mg*

93. Cinnamon Pistachio-Orange Smoothie

Preparation time: 5 minutes

Cooking time: 01 minutes

Serving: 2

Difficulty level: Easy

Ingredients

- 1/2 cup plain whole-milk Greek yogurt (approx. 123g / 4.3 oz US / 0.27 lb US)
- 1/2 cup unsweetened almond milk (approx. 120ml / 4 fl oz US)
- Zest and juice of 1 clementine or 1/2 orange (zest approx. 1 tsp; juice approx. 2 tbsp)
- 1 tbsp extra-virgin olive oil or MCT oil (approx. 14g / 0.5 oz US / 0.03 lb US)
- 1 tbsp shelled pistachios, coarsely chopped (approx. 14g / 0.5 oz US / 0.03 lb US)
- 1 to 2 tsp monk fruit extract or stevia (optional) (approx. 4-8g / 0.14-0.28 oz US / 0.008-0.017 lb US)
- 1/4 to 1/2 tsp ground allspice (approx. 0.5-1g / 0.017-0.035 oz US / 0.0011-0.0022 lb US)
- 1/4 tsp ground cinnamon (approx. 0.5g / 0.017 oz US / 0.0011 lb US)
- 1/4 tsp vanilla extract (approx. 1.2ml / 0.04 fl oz US)

Directions:

1. In a blender, combine the plain whole-milk Greek yogurt, unsweetened almond milk, zest and juice of a clementine or orange, extra-virgin olive oil or MCT oil, shelled pistachios, monk fruit extract or stevia (if using), ground allspice, ground cinnamon, and vanilla extract.
2. Blend until the mixture achieves a creamy and smooth consistency.
3. Pour the smoothie into serving glasses.

Nutritional information

- *Calories: 342*
- *Fat: 23g*
- *Sodium: 144mg*
- *Carbohydrates: 30g*
- *Fiber: 3g*
- *Protein: 7g*

94. Ginger-Pear Smoothie

Preparation time: 5 minutes

Cooking time: 0 minutes

Serving: 2

Difficulty level: Medium

Ingredients

- 1 pear, cored and quartered (approx. 178g / 6.3 oz US / 0.39 lb US); 1/2 fennel bulb (approx. 100g / 3.5 oz US / 0.22 lb US); 1 thin slice of fresh ginger (approx. 2g / 0.07 oz US / 0.004 lb US)
- 1 cup packed spinach (approx. 30g / 1 oz US / 0.06 lb US)
- 1/2 cucumber, peeled if wax-coated or not organic (approx. 150g / 5.3 oz US / 0.33 lb US); 1/2 cup water (approx. 120ml / 4 fl oz US); Ice (optional)

Directions:

1. Combine the pear, fennel bulb, fresh ginger, spinach, cucumber, and water in a blender.
2. If desired, add ice for texture.
3. Blend the mixture until it reaches a creamy and smooth consistency.
4. Pour the smoothie into serving glasses.

Nutritional information

- *Calories: 108*
- *Fat: 1g*
- *Sodium: 89mg*
- *Carbohydrates: 25g*
- *Protein: 4g*

95. Dandelion and Beet Greens Detox Smoothie

Preparation time: 5 minutes

Cooking time: 0 minutes

Serving: 2

Difficulty level: Easy

Ingredients

- 6 ice cubes (optional for texture)
- 1 cup almond milk (240ml / 8.45 fl oz US)
- 2 tbsp almond butter (32g / 1.13 oz US)
- 1 medium banana, peeled and frozen (118g / 4.16 oz US)
- 1 cup dandelion greens (55g / 1.94 oz US)
- 1 cup beet greens (38g / 1.34 oz US)

Directions:

1. Place the ice cubes, almond milk, almond butter, banana, dandelion greens, and beet greens into a blender.
2. Blend the mixture until it achieves a smooth and creamy consistency.
3. Pour the smoothie into glasses and serve immediately.

Nutritional information

- *Calories: 97.2*
- *Carbohydrates: 31.1g*
- *Protein: 5.9g*
- *Fat: 10.8g*
- *Sodium: 186mg*

96. Beans, Peaches, and Greens Smoothie

Preparation time: 5 minutes

Cooking time: 0 minutes

Serving: 2

Difficulty level: Easy

> ### Ingredients
>
> - Pinch of nutmeg (less than 0.1g / less than 0.0035 oz US)
> - 1/8 tsp cinnamon (0.25g / 0.0088 oz US)
> - 1/4 cup canned white beans, rinsed and drained well (about 45g / 1.59 oz US)
> - 1 cup frozen peaches (154g / 5.43 oz US)
> - 1 cup almond milk (240ml / 8.45 fl oz US)
> - 1/4 cup quick-cooking oats (21.25g / 0.75 oz US)
> - 1 cup packed lettuce (any kind) (70g / 2.47 oz US)
> - 1/4 cup Italian parsley (15g / 0.53 oz US)
> - 6 cubes of ice (optional for texture)

Directions:

1. Combine the nutmeg, cinnamon, white beans, frozen peaches, almond milk, oats, lettuce, parsley, and ice cubes in a blender.
2. Blend the mixture until it reaches a smooth and creamy consistency.
3. Pour the smoothie into glasses and serve immediately.

Nutritional information

- *Calories: 231.8*
- *Carbohydrates: 50g*
- *Protein: 3g*
- *Fat: 2.2g*
- *Sodium: 99mg*

97. Simple Almond Butter-Banana Smoothie

Preparation time: 3 minutes

Cooking time: 0 minutes

Serving: 2

Difficulty level: Easy

> ### Ingredients
>
> - 1 medium frozen banana, chopped (118g / 4.16 oz US)
> - 3/4 cup unsweetened almond milk (180ml / 6.09 fl oz US)
> - 1 tbsp raw, unsalted almond butter (16g / 0.56 oz US)
> - 1/4 cup water (59ml / 2 fl oz US)
> - 1 1/2 tbsp unsweetened cocoa powder (7.5g / 0.26 oz US)
> - 1/8 tsp ground cinnamon (0.25g / 0.0088 oz US)
> - 3 drops almond extract (approx. 0.15ml / 0.005 fl oz US)
> - 3–4 ice cubes (optional for texture)
> - Sprig of fresh mint for garnish (0.2g / 0.007 oz US)

Directions:

1. Combine the banana, almond milk, almond butter, water, cocoa powder, cinnamon, almond extract, and ice cubes in a blender.
2. Blend on high speed until the mixture is smooth, which should take about 1 minute.
3. For a thicker consistency, add additional ice cubes and blend again.
4. Pour the smoothie into two glasses and garnish with a sprig of fresh mint.
5. Serve immediately and enjoy.

Nutritional information

- *Calories: 257*
- *Fat: 10g*
- *Sodium: 84mg*
- *Carbohydrates: 43g*
- *Protein: 4g*

4.10 Snack Time: Heart-Healthy Options

98. Cannellini Bean Hummus

Preparation time: 10 minutes

Cooking time: 0 minutes

Serving: 2

Difficulty level: Easy

Ingredients

- 30 oz can cannellini beans, drained and rinsed (850g / 29.98 oz US)
- 1/4 cup olive oil (59ml / 2 fl oz US)
- 1/8 tsp chili powder (0.6ml / 0.02 fl oz US)
- 1 tsp garlic powder (2.8g / 0.1 oz US)
- 1 tsp cumin powder (2.1g / 0.07 oz US)
- 3 tbsp fresh lemon juice (44ml / 1.5 fl oz US)
- 1/4 cup water (59ml / 2 fl oz US)
- 1/2 tbsp salt (7g / 0.2 oz US)

Directions:

1. Place the cannellini beans, olive oil, chili powder, garlic powder, cumin powder, lemon juice, water, and a reduced amount of salt (recommend 1/4 to 1/2 teaspoon) into a food processor.
2. Process the mixture until it reaches the desired consistency.
3. Serve immediately or store in the refrigerator for later use. Enjoy with vegetables or whole-grain crackers.

Nutritional information

- *Fat: 3.2g*
- *Carbohydrates: 9g*
- *Protein: 3.1g*

⚠ The original recipe calls for a tablespoon of salt, which is significantly high, especially for individuals managing heart conditions that require low sodium intake. It is recommended to reduce the salt to 1/4 to 1/2 teaspoon to align with heart-healthy dietary guidelines. Olive oil and cannellini beans are good sources of healthy fats and fiber, respectively, which are beneficial for heart health.

99. Guacamole with Jicama

Preparation time: 5 minutes

Cooking time: 0 minutes

Serving: 2

Difficulty level: Medium

Ingredients

- 1 avocado, cut into cubes (about 150g / 5.3 oz US)
- Juice of 1/2 lime (approximately 15ml / 0.5 fl oz US)
- 2 tbsp finely chopped shallots (about 15g / 0.5 oz US)
- 2 tbsp chopped fresh parsley (about 7.6g / 0.3 oz US)
- 1 garlic clove, minced (about 3g / 0.1 oz US)
- 1/4 tsp salt (1.5g / 0.05 oz US) — Consider reducing or omitting for heart health.
- 1 cup sliced jicama (about 120g / 4.2 oz US)

Directions:

1. In a small bowl, combine the avocado, lime juice, shallots, parsley, garlic, and a pinch of salt (if using).
2. Mash the ingredients together with a fork to your desired consistency.
3. Serve the guacamole with jicama slices for dipping.

Nutritional information

- *Fat: 5g*
- *Sodium: 77mg*
- *Carbohydrates: 8g*
- *Protein: 1g*

⚠ The inclusion of salt in this recipe should be approached with caution for individuals with heart conditions, particularly those requiring sodium restriction. It is advisable to reduce or eliminate the added salt. Avocado is a heart-healthy fruit rich in monounsaturated fats, which can be beneficial for heart health when consumed in moderation. Jicama provides a low-calorie, high-fiber dipping option, which is also favorable for heart health

100. Homemade Kale Chips

Preparation time: 20 minutes

Cooking time: 20 minutes

Serving: 2

Difficulty level: Easy

Ingredients

- 1 bunch kale, washed, dried, ribs removed, cut into 2-inch strips (approximately 200g / 7 oz US)
- 2 tbsp extra-virgin olive oil (30ml / 1 fl oz US)
- 1 tsp sea salt (5g / 0.18 oz US) — Consider reducing for heart health.

Directions:

1. Preheat your oven to 275°F (135°C).
2. In a large bowl, gently massage the kale with olive oil until each piece is lightly coated.
3. Arrange the kale in a single layer on a baking sheet, ensuring the pieces do not overlap.
4. Lightly sprinkle the kale with sea salt, using less if sodium intake is a concern.
5. Bake in the preheated oven for approximately 20 minutes or until the kale is crisp, turning halfway through to ensure even crispness.
6. Allow the chips to cool slightly before serving to enhance the crisp texture.

Nutritional information

- *Calories: 93 (This may vary depending on the size of the kale bunch.)*
- *Fat: 7g*
- *Sodium: 497mg*
- *Carbohydrates: 7g*
- *Protein: 2g*

⚠ The sodium content in this recipe may be higher than recommended for individuals with heart conditions. It is advisable to reduce or eliminate the added salt to lower the sodium content. Olive oil is a source of monounsaturated fats, which are considered heart-healthy when consumed in moderation. Kale is rich in antioxidants and fiber, which are beneficial for cardiovascular health.

101. Cucumber Caprese Snack Boxes

Preparation time: 15 minutes

Cooking time: 0 minutes

Serving: 2

Difficulty level: Medium

Ingredients

For each snack box (total of 4 boxes):

- 1/4 cup cherry tomatoes (about 37g / 1.3 oz)
- 1/2 medium Kirby cucumber, halved lengthwise and cut into 1/2-inch bites (approximately 50g / 1.8 oz)
- 1/4 cup fresh mozzarella pearls (about 30g / 1 oz)
- 1/4 cup pitted Kalamata olives (about 33g / 1.2 oz)
- 1 tbsp red pepper flakes (about 7g / 0.25 oz) — Consider reducing for heart health.
- 1 tbsp dried basil (about 2g / 0.07 oz)

Directions:

1. In a small, airtight container, layer the cherry tomatoes, cucumber bites, mozzarella pearls, and Kalamata olives.

2. Season with red pepper flakes and dried basil to taste, being mindful of the potential for red pepper flakes to be spicy.

3. Assemble three additional snack boxes using the same method.

4. Store the containers in the refrigerator, maintaining airtight conditions to preserve freshness for up to four days.

Nutritional information

- *Calories: 139 (per snack box)*
- *Fat: 9g*
- *Sodium: 383mg — This is a moderate amount. Those with heart conditions should monitor sodium intake.*
- *Carbohydrates: 10g*
- *Protein: 7g*

⚠ The sodium content in this recipe may be of concern for individuals with heart conditions, particularly if consumed frequently. The use of Kalamata olives and mozzarella contributes to the sodium content; choosing lower-sodium alternatives or reducing the portion size could be beneficial.

102. Mexican Street Snack

Preparation time: 15 minutes

Cooking time: 0 minutes

Serving: 2

Difficulty level: Easy

Ingredients

- 1 medium jicama, peeled and cut into 1/2-by-3-inch-long matchsticks (approximately 1 lb or 453.6g)
- Juice of 1 lime (about 2 tablespoons or 30ml)
- 1 tsp chili powder (about 2.6g) — Consider reducing for heart health.
- Pinch of salt (less than 1/4 tsp or 1.5g) — Use sparingly for heart health.
- 2 medium mangos, cut into 1/4-inch wedges (each mango approximately 200g without refuse)

Directions:

1. In a mixing bowl, combine the jicama sticks and mango wedges.
2. Drizzle with fresh lime juice, and sprinkle with chili powder and a pinch of salt. Toss the ingredients to ensure an even coating.
3. The mixture can be stored in an airtight container and refrigerated, maintaining its quality for up to four days.

Nutritional information

- *Calories: 112 (per serving)*
- *Fat: 1g*
- *Sodium: 37mg — This is a low amount, suitable for those monitoring sodium intake for heart health.*
- *Carbohydrates: 27g*
- *Protein: 2g*

---

103. Butternut Squash Fries

Preparation time: 5 minutes

Cooking time: 20 minutes

Serving: 2

Difficulty level: Medium

Ingredients

- 2 butternut squash (approximately 2-3 lbs or 907g-1.36kg each)
- 2 tbsp olive oil (30ml)
- 2 tbsp thyme (about 6g, fresh if possible)
- 2 tbsp rosemary (about 3.5g, fresh if possible)
- 1/2 tsp salt (2.5g) — Consider reducing for heart health.
- Cooking spray (preferably olive oil-based)

Directions:

1. Preheat the oven to 425°F (220°C).
2. Coat a baking sheet with cooking spray.
3. Peel the butternut squash and cut into fry-shaped pieces.
4. In a bowl, combine the squash fries with olive oil, thyme, rosemary, and salt, ensuring an even coat.
5. Arrange the fries on the prepared baking sheet in a single layer.
6. Bake in the preheated oven for 10 minutes, then remove and gently toss the fries.
7. Please return to the oven and continue baking for an additional 10 minutes or until they are golden and crisp.
8. Serve immediately.

Nutritional information

- *Calories: 62 (per serving)*
- *Fat: 2g*
- *Sodium: 2.5g — This is a moderate amount; consider reducing it to 1/4 tsp or 1.25g for heart health.*
- *Carbohydrates: 11g*

Chapter #5: A 28-Day Heart-Healthy Meal Plan

Week 1: Initiating a Heart-Healthy Regimen

Days	Breakfast	Lunch	Dinner	Snack/Dessert
1	Zucchini stuffed breakfast	Coconut and almond rice with berries	Vegan fajita bowl with cabbage rice	Banana strawberry muffins
2	Green scrambled eggs	Tabouli salad	Curried shrimp salad in a papaya	Ricotta stuffed peaches
3	Roasted pepper frittata	Broccoli slaw	Lentils with rice and onions	Ricotta stuffed peaches
4	Spinach burrito	Grilled vegetable and pineapple salad	Healthy chicken pasta salad	Sweet potato and pumpkin pie
5	Trail hot cereal	Asparagus pasta	Black bean spread with maple syrup	Apple-berry cobbler
6	Breakfast cereal with apples and raisins	Root vegetable curry	Veggie burger with spice medley	Fruit compote
7	Greek eggs with potatoes	Cauliflower-cream pasta with mint	Potato and vegetable casserole	Creamy, delicious farro

Week 2: Delving Deeper into Nutritional Wellness

Days	Breakfast	Lunch	Dinner	Snack/Dessert
8	Delicious breakfast barley	Broccoli rice casserole	Cabbage pilaf	Brown rice pudding
9	Peanut butter oats	Spiced eggplant fritters	Roasted potatoes with herbs	Watermelon wedges with lemon
10	Quark cucumber toast	Seafood with sundried tomatoes and pasta	Roasted red pepper hummus	Cherry stew
11	Zucchini stuffed breakfast	Vegetable kabobs	Perfect sweet potatoes	Nutritious roasted chickpeas
12	Green scrambled eggs	Salmon, spinach, and tomato lasagna	Vegetarian Bolognese	Crispy carrot fries
13	Roasted pepper frittata	Cod cauliflower chowder	Steamed salmon teriyaki	Cannellini bean hummus
14	Spinach burrito	Grilled pork fajitas	Seafood tomato stew	Guacamole with jicama

Week 3: Celebrating Dietary Diversity

Days	Breakfast	Lunch	Dinner	Snack/Dessert
15	Trail hot cereal	Spicy beef kebabs	Grilled Vegetable and Pineapple Salad	Homemade kale chips
16	Breakfast cereal with apples and raisins	Roasted salmon with maple-balsamic glaze	Herbed Smashed Potatoes with Garlic	Cucumber Caprese snack boxes
17	Greek eggs with potatoes	Beef Stroganoff	Root Vegetable Curry	Mexican street snack
18	Delicious breakfast barley	Chicken fajitas	Baked salmon with fennel	Butternut squash fries
19				
20	Peanut butter oats	Flounder with tomatoes	Miso-glazed tuna	Strawberry cocoa smoothie
21	Quark cucumber toast	Salmon sage bake	Curried pork tenderloin in apple cider	Peanut strawberry smoothie

Week 4: Reinforcing Heart-Healthy Habits

Days	Breakfast	Lunch	Dinner	Snack/Dessert
22	Strawberry cocoa smoothie	Shish kabob	Spicy chili salmon	Simple almond butter-banana smoothie
23	Peanut strawberry smoothie	Healthy turkey chili	Mix of mackerel and orange	Beans, peaches, and greens smoothie
24	Apple tart smoothie	Beef and vegetable kebabs	Chicken with orzo and lemon	Banana strawberry muffins
25	Green mango smoothie	Pasta creole style	Salmon with marinade	Ricotta stuffed peaches
26	Cinnamon pistachio-orange smoothie	Jerk seasoned meat loaves	Grilled pork fajitas	Sweet potato and pumpkin pie
27	Ginger-pear smoothie	Crispy cashew fish sticks	Cod with citrus salad	Fruit compote
28	Dandelion and beet greens detox smoothie	Seafood with sundried tomatoes and pasta	Chicken salad with oranges	Creamy, delicious farro

Chapter 6

The Heart Healthy Shopping List

FRESH VEGETABLES & FRUIT

Apple; Oranges; Berries; Pears; Cayenne peppers; Tomatoes
Squash cauliflower; Zucchini broccoli; Celery Kale; Pak choy
Grapes; Eggplant; Asparagus; Berries in red Blackberries
Broccoli; Cabbage; Spinach; Chard (Swiss chard)
Tomatoes in red; Tomatoes that are yellow
Vegetables with green leaves; Vegetables, raw; Carrots

DAIRY & DAIRY SUBSTITUTES

Dairy products are high in calcium.
Choose low-fat or nonfat foods instead of cream.
Low-fat or nonfat buttermilk; Nonfat or reduced-fat cheese;
Nonfat cottage cheese or ricotta cheese;
Nonfat cream cheese; Milk made from almonds;
Skimmed milk; Nonfat sour cream; Nonfat yogurt; Tofu milk
Choose unsweetened foods and avoid foods with added sugar.

MEAT, POULTRY, FISH, AND MEAT ALTERNATIVES

Beef, lean cuts, ground round, or sirloin
Skinless and boneless chicken or turkey breasts and tenders
Ground chicken or turkey
Fish such as herring, mackerel, salmon, trout, and tuna
Seitan; Tofu made from Tempeh

SPICES

Basil, The bay leaves, The spice of black pepper, Cumin seeds
Cayenne, Chili flakes, Five-spice powder from China
Cinnamon, Cloves, Coriander, Curry powder with cumin
Dill, Roasted garlic powder, Ginger Seasoning from Italy
Marjoram, Mint, Nutmeg, The powdered onion, Oregano
Paprika and parsley, Flakes of red pepper, Rosemary
Thyme, Seasonings with no sodium

COOKING OILS AND FATS

Transfat-free margarine
Cooking sprays that are low in fat,
Olive and canola oils
Applesauce and fruit puree can be used
as fat substitutes in baking

FOODS THAT HAVE BEEN FROZEN

Strawberries, raspberries,
and blueberries
have no added sugar
Soybeans, Soup of vegetables
with no added sodium or sugar

PANTRY ESSENTIALS

Barley; Reduced-sodium canned beans: beans in various cans
Dried beans: select your favorite beans.
Broth, chicken, beef, or vegetable broth with reduced sodium
Wholegrain cereal; Cornmeal; Flaxseed, Whole wheat flour
Wheat berries, couscous, polenta, millet, bulgur, and quinoa
Bran of oats, Tomato sauce, Low-fat or fat-free rolled, steel-cut oats
Pasta: fettuccini, lasagna, spaghetti, fusilli, spiral, elbow macaroni,
and ravioli made from whole wheat, spelt, or Kamut.
Brown, wild, and brown basmati rice, Low-sodium soups
Tofu flour, Reduced-sodium tomatoes, whole or diced,
Refried beans that are vegetarian or low in fat
Barbecue sauce, low-sodium Ketchup,
reduced-sodium Mayonnaise, reduced-fat or non-fat cheese
Whole grain, honey, Dijon, and yellow mustard, Reduced-sodium soy sauce
Vinegar includes rice, red wine, balsamic, apple cider, and raspberry.

OTHER

Snacks include almonds, walnuts, sunflower seeds, and sesame seeds.
Fruits that have been dried. Tortillas, pitas, and wholegrain bread.
Wholegrain crackers with no trans-fat. Brown rice cakes or popcorn cakes.
Baked popcorn tortilla chips with no trans fats.
Pretzels, wholegrain.
.Syrup made from brown rice
Agave, Sweetener, low-carbohydrate

Chapter 7

Measurement Conversion Table

COOKING CONVERSION CHART

Measurement

CUP	ONCES	MILLILITERS	TABLESPOONS
8 cup	64 oz	1895 ml	128
6 cup	48 oz	1420 ml	96
5 cup	40 oz	1180 ml	80
4 cup	32 oz	960 ml	64
2 cup	16 oz	480 ml	32
1 cup	8 oz	240 ml	16
3/4 cup	6 oz	177 ml	12
2/3 cup	5 oz	158 ml	11
1/2 cup	4 oz	118 ml	8
3/8 cup	3 oz	90 ml	6
1/3 cup	2.5 oz	79 ml	5.5
1/4 cup	2 oz	59 ml	4
1/8 cup	1 oz	30 ml	3
1/16 cup	1/2 oz	15 ml	1

Temperature

FAHRENHEIT	CELSIUS
100 °F	37 °C
150 °F	65 °C
200 °F	93 °C
250 °F	121 °C
300 °F	150 °C
325 °F	160 °C
350 °F	180 °C
375 °F	190 °C
400 °F	200 °C
425 °F	220 °C
450 °F	230 °C
500 °F	260 °C
525 °F	274 °C
550 °F	288 °C

Weight

IMPERIAL	METRIC
1/2 oz	15 g
1 oz	29 g
2 oz	57 g
3 oz	85 g
4 oz	113 g
5 oz	141 g
6 oz	170 g
8 oz	227 g
10 oz	283 g
12 oz	340 g
13 oz	369 g
14 oz	397 g
15 oz	425 g
1 lb	453 g

Thank You!

Thank you for choosing to spend your valuable time exploring Cardiovascular Prevention Guide with us. We genuinely hope that the information and insights provided within these pages have enriched your understanding and will guide you in your journey towards improved health and well-being.

One small request, if we may: your opinions matter enormously, not just to us but also to potential future readers. If you found value in this book, would you be so kind as to share your thoughts in a **quick review**? Your insights and experiences can help others who are interested in exploring the world of cardiovascular well-being, offering comprehensive insights into maintaining a healthy heart.

To write a few words about what you liked, what you learned, or how you plan to apply this knowledge, would be immensely appreciated.

Simply click the link or scan the QR code below to leave your review:

https://qrco.de/becRoE

SCAN ME

And remember, each review is a step towards helping those aspiring to prioritize and enhance their overall cardiovascular well-being.

You're amazing for being part of this journey!

To your health and well-being,

Rose and Paul

✻ HERE IS YOU FREE GIFT!

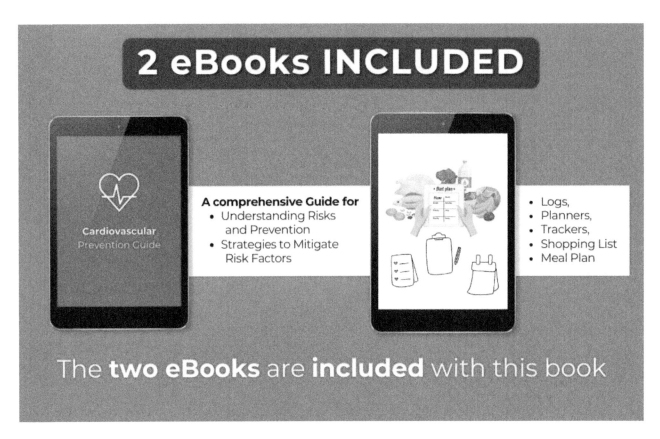

👇 SCAN HERE TO DOWNLOAD IT

Conclusion

As we bring this journey through our heart-healthy diet cookbook to a close, it's time to reflect on the significant strides we've made. Embracing a heart-healthy diet is more than a dietary choice; it's a commitment to a life brimming with vitality and joy. This cookbook has been crafted to shatter the myth that healthy eating is monotonous or limiting, showcasing instead how it can be both simple and delicious.

At the heart of this diet are fresh vegetables, including leafy greens, beans, spinach, broccoli, Brussels sprouts, and tomatoes. These nutrient-rich foods are perfectly paired with a variety of fresh fruits like apples, oranges, and pears, alongside legumes, whole grains, seafood, and premium dairy products. The focus is on minimizing intake of high-carbohydrate, high-fat, and high-sodium foods, which are known culprits in heart-related health issues.

But a heart-healthy lifestyle extends beyond what's on your plate. Regular physical activity and staying hydrated are key pillars of maintaining a healthy heart. The diet's foundation of healthy fats, vitamins, minerals, and proteins work in harmony to bolster your overall health.

Moderation is also key, particularly when it comes to salt and sugar intake. Excessive sodium is a major risk factor for hypertension, a leading cause of heart disease. While the recipes in this cookbook offer a fantastic starting point, consulting with a healthcare professional is advisable before making significant dietary changes, especially for those with existing health conditions.

Incorporating the recipes and foods from this cookbook into your daily life is a proactive step towards enhancing your cardiovascular health and reducing the risk of heart disease. This cookbook is more than a collection of recipes; it's a guide to a healthier heart and a more joyful life.

The mindset with which you approach this dietary change is crucial. Stay motivated and find joy in exploring new, heart-healthy culinary delights. Mindful eating, the practice of being fully present and savoring each meal, not only enriches the eating experience but also fosters a deeper appreciation for the nourishing foods you consume.

As you continue on this heart-healthy journey, remember that each meal is an opportunity to nurture your heart and body. Armed with the knowledge and recipes from this cookbook, you're well-equipped to make heart-healthy eating an enjoyable and integral part of your life. Here's to your health and happiness – wishing you all the best on this rewarding journey!

Printed in Great Britain
by Amazon

37974262R00064